EXTERNAL EYE DISEASE: A COLOUR ATLAS

For Churchill Livingstone

Publisher: Mike Parkinson
Editorial Co-ordination: Editorial Resources Unit
Copy Editor: Paul Singleton
Production Controller: Lesley W. Small
Design: Design Resources Unit
Sales Promotion Executive: Marion Pollock

EXTERNAL EYE DISEASE: A COLOUR ATLAS

Mark T. Watts
MB ChB FRCS FCOphth
Senior Registrar in Ophthalmology, Royal Hallamshire Hospital, Sheffield, UK

Michael E. Nelson
MB ChB FRCS FCOphth
Consultant Ophthalmologist, Royal Hallamshire Hospital, Sheffield, UK

FOREWORD BY
Michael Roper-Hall
ChM MB ChB FRCS FCOphth DOMS

CHURCHILL LIVINGSTONE
EDINBURGH LONDON MADRID
MELBOURNE NEW YORK AND TOKYO
1992

CHURCHILL LIVINGSTONE
Medical Division of Longman Group UK Limited

Distributed in the United States of America by Churchill Livingstone Inc., 650 Avenue of the Americas, New York, N.Y. 10011, and by associated companies, branches and representatives throughout the world.

First published 1992

ISBN 0-443-04446-5

British Library Cataloguing in Publication Data
A catalogue record for this book is available from the British Library.

Library of Congress Cataloging in Publication Data
Watts, Mark T.

External eye disease : a colour atlas / Mark T. Watts and Michael E. Nelson; foreword by Michael Roper-Hall.

p. cm.

Includes index.

ISBN 0-443-04446-5

1. Anterior segment (Eye) — Diseases — Atlases.
2. Eyelids — Diseases — Atlases.

[DNLM: 1. Eye Diseases — diagnosis — atlases.
2. Eye Diseases — pathology — atlases. 3. Eye Diseases — therapy — atlases. WW 17 W352e]

RE71.W38 1992

617.7′7 — dc20 91-34183

CIP

The publisher's policy is to use **paper manufactured from sustainable forests**

Printed in Hong Kong
CTPS/01

FOREWORD

It is a pleasure to write this Foreword, as I know the authors and the care they have taken in the preparation of the text and illustrations. They both have a particular interest in external eye disease and have a wealth of clinical material available to them. They do not claim their book to be comprehensive, but it is extensive and covers the great majority of conditions seen in a year of out-patient attendances.

The book is concise and easy to read, using current terminology correctly and avoiding jargon. It includes recent advances in the understanding and treatment of diseases of the external eye. The emphasis is on diagnosis, with a general indication of current therapy and diagrammatic depiction of surgery, when this is appropriate. The authors refer in the bibliographies to more substantial texts. Primarily intended as a 'pattern recognition' book, it will be particularly useful to trainees who are preparing for examinations. It should also be very useful for clinical reference by those faced with the primary consultation who have not seen the conditions before, because a written description cannot match the impact of high quality colour illustrations. These have been carefully placed alongside the relevant text.

The quality of this book should be appreciated by a wide readership.

1992 **M. J. R.-H.**

ACKNOWLEDGEMENTS

We are indebted to Christopher Mody, ophthalmic photographer at the Royal Hallamshire Hospital, who has not only taken a large proportion of the photographs, but also drawn the accompanying line diagrams. We would also like to thank Dr Andy Parsons, who prepared the histological sections. A number of contributors, who are acknowledged in the text, have kindly allowed us to use their photographs, for which we are most grateful.

M. T. W.
M. E. N.

PREFACE

The purpose of this atlas is to provide principally a photographic account of external eye disease, and the accompanying text gives a brief summary of the conditions and their management. It is not intended as a detailed review of all aspects of external eye disease. We have tried to highlight the systemic features of conditions where appropriate.

External Eye Disease: A Colour Atlas is intended primarily for general ophthalmologists and ophthalmologists in training, but should also prove of interest to physicians in associated fields, such as dermatology and rheumatology, as well as to optometrists in clinical practice.

Sheffield
1992

M. T. W.
M. E. N.

CONTENTS

SECTION 2
THE CONJUNCTIVA 29

SECTION 3
THE CORNEA 63

1
THE EYELIDS

ANATOMY

Both upper (Fig. 1.1.1) and lower (Fig. 1.1.2) lids consist of an anterior and posterior lamella. Along the lid margin, which is approximately 2 mm thick, runs a thin 'grey line' marking the division between the two lamellae, and where the lids can be split (Fig. 1.1.3).

The anterior lamella contains the eyelashes and lash follicles, orbicularis muscle, and vascular supply to the lid. The lower lid has a single palpebral artery, which runs parallel to the lid margin, in front of the tarsal plate. The upper lid has two such arteries, one of which runs in front of, and the other just above, the tarsal plate. The sebaceous glands of Zeiss are attached to the eyelash follicles, and the glands of Moll drain either into these glands, or separately in between the lashes.

The posterior lamella contains the tarsal plate lined on the inner surface by conjunctiva. The tarsal plate consists of dense fibrous tissue. Meibomian glands, which are modified sebaceous glands, are situated within it and drain onto the lid margin. All the glands of the lids contribute to the superficial lipid layer of the tear film. The tarsal plates provide rigidity to the lids, and give them shape. The medial and lateral canthal tendons are fibrous extensions at the sides of the tarsal plates which are attached to the orbital margin. Muscles control the position of both tarsal plates. In the lower lids these are termed the lower lid retractors. They arise from the sheath of the inferior rectus muscle and attach to the tarsal plate. The muscles of the upper lid comprise the levator palpebrae superioris and Müller's muscle which arise from a common origin at the apex of the orbit. The tendon of the levator muscle inserts between the orbicularis fibres to create the skin crease. A fibrous orbital septum separates the orbital fat from the orbicularis muscle. It arises from the bony margins of the orbit, and inserts into the retractors or levator musculature.

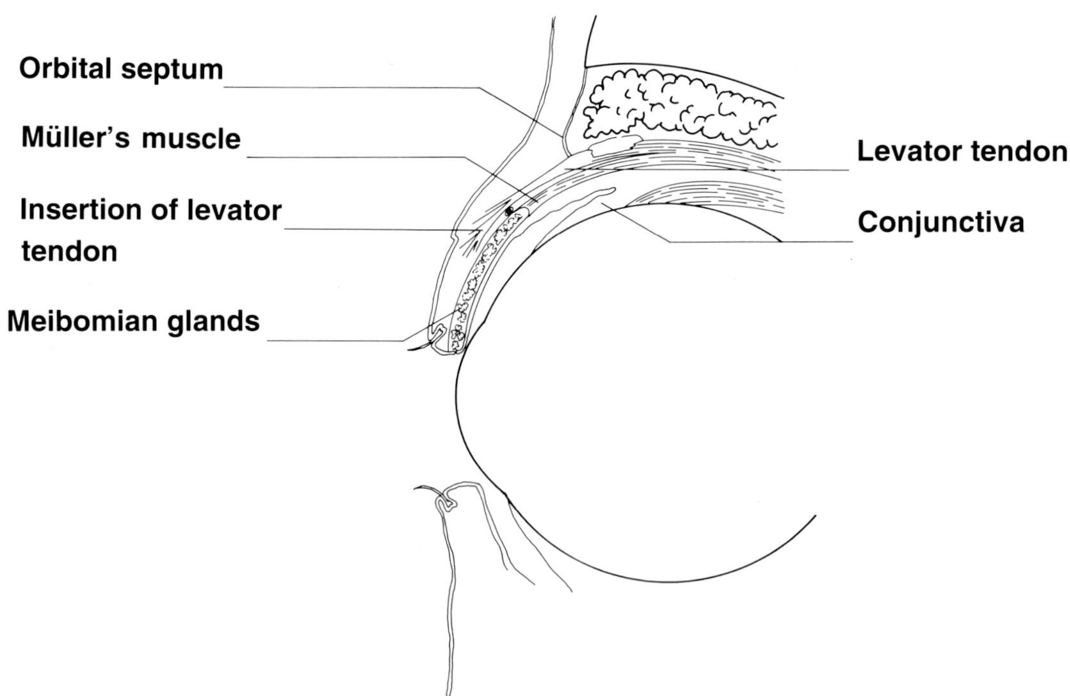

Fig. 1.1.1 The upper eyelid.

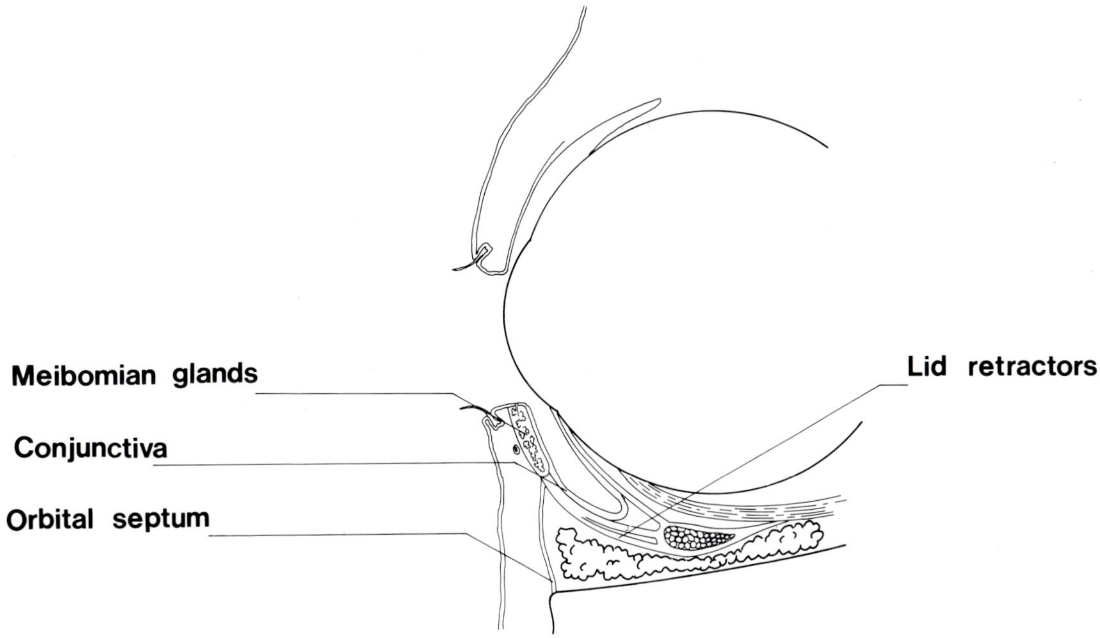

Fig. 1.1.2 The lower eyelid.

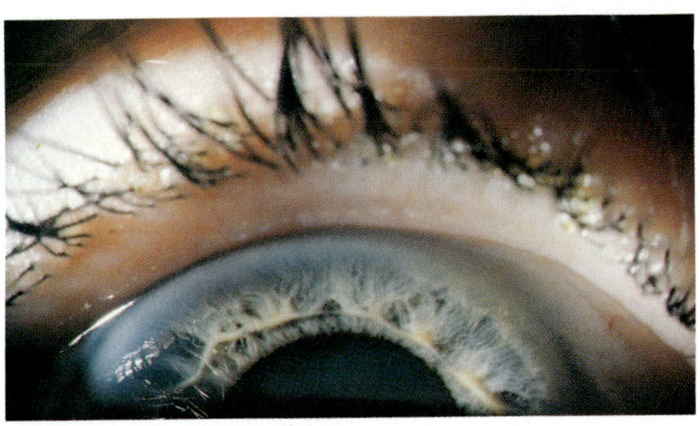

Fig. 1.1.3 The grey line.

MALPOSITIONS

Normal eyelid position is dependent on the rigidity provided by the tarsal plate, adequate tone in the musculature supporting the lids, and the attachment and integrity of the canthal tendons. Failure of any of these elements may lead to malposition, and consequent exposure or abrasion of the cornea.

Ectropion

Involutional

Ectropion is most commonly due to involutional changes leading to laxity of the musculature and tendons of the lids. Atrophy of orbital fat tissue and the resultant enophthalmos often exacerbate the situation. Chronic exposure of the conjunctiva caused by the ectropion leads to metaplasia of the conjunctival goblet cells, and keratinization of the stratified squamous epithelium (Fig. 1.2.1). This abrasive surface readily irritates the globe, predisposing to corneal ulceration and infection.

Treatment involves horizontal shortening of the lid, often in conjunction with removal of some lid skin, if this too is excessively lax. Inverting sutures (Quickert–Rathbun) (Fig. 1.2.2) can help rotate the lid margin inwards. Ectropion may be localized to one segment of the lid. Medial ectropion everts the punctum away from the tear lake, and leads to epiphora (Fig. 1.2.3). This may be treated by cautery or resection of tissue of the posterior lamella of the lid below the canaliculus, so as to invert the punctum.

Cicatricial

Ectropion may also be caused by cicatrization of the lid skin most commonly following burns, excessive surgical resection or radiotherapy (Fig. 1.2.4). If of a very minor degree, regular massage of the lid skin using a lubricant cream, may achieve resolution. More severe scarring necessitates surgical correction. A block resection of lid margin and tarsal plate can often satisfactorily reposition mild ectropion. Techniques aimed at repositioning the remaining skin (e.g. Z-plasty: Fig. 1.2.5a and b), or full-thickness skin grafting are required for more severe cicatrization or tissue loss. The best donor sites for such grafts are the post-auricular region and the upper eyelid skin.

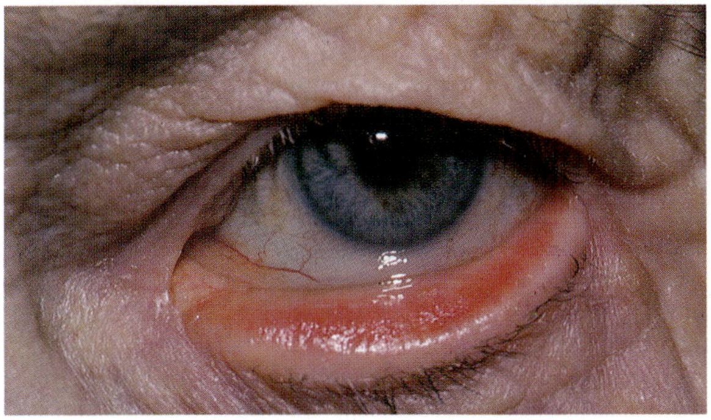

Fig. 1.2.1 Conjunctival keratinization secondary to involutional ectropion.

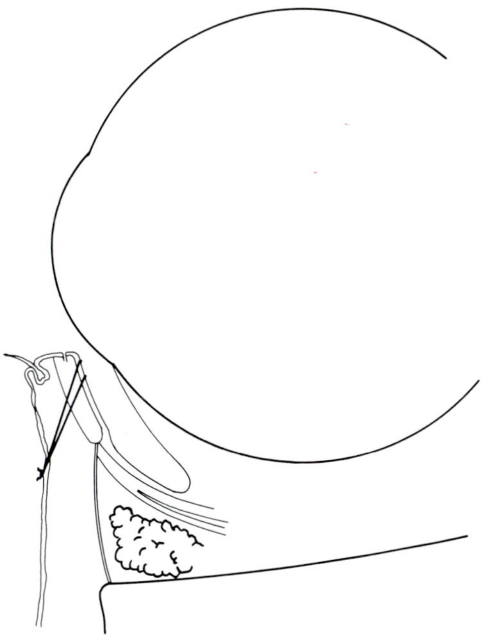

Fig. 1.2.2 Quickert–Rathbun sutures to invert the lower lid.

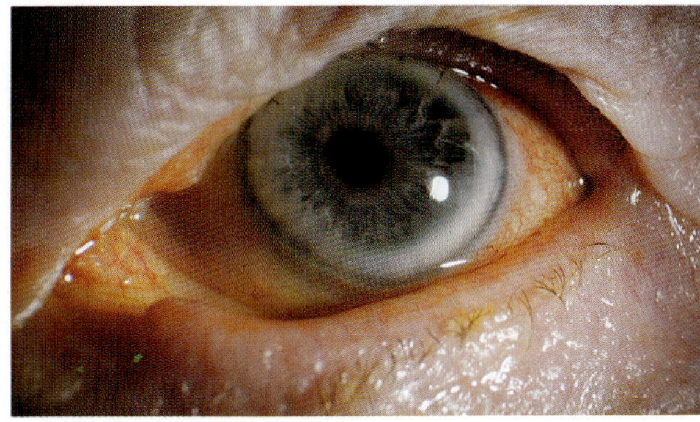

Fig. 1.2.3 Medial ectropion.

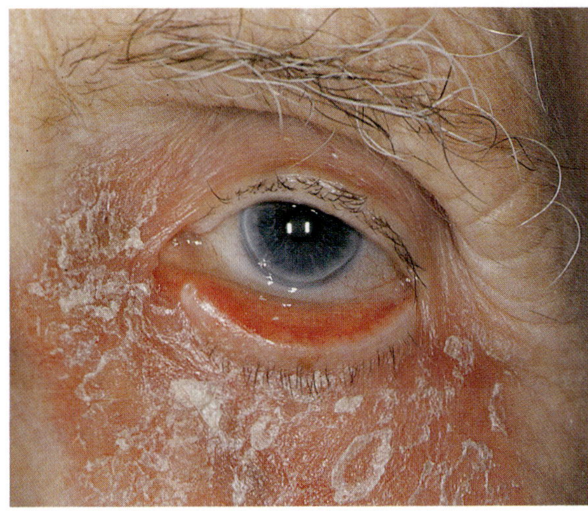

Fig. 1.2.4 Cicatricial ectropion.

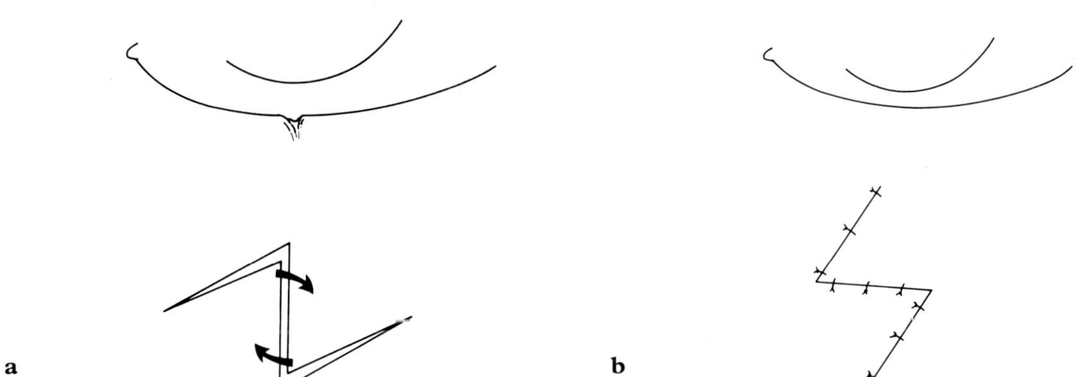

Fig. 1.2.5 The use of Z-plasty to relieve vertical skin tension due to cicatrization: before (**a**) and after (**b**).

Paralytic

Damage to the facial nerve leads to paralytic ectropion and failure of adequate lid closure (Fig. 1.2.6) because of paralysis of orbicularis musculature. If the weakness is likely to recover, as for example in Bell's palsy or following contusion of the nerve during neurosurgery, then a temporary lateral tarsorrhaphy (Fig. 1.2.7) normally affords good protection to the cornea. This can be opened when normal orbicularis tone has been re-established. Complete and permanent facial nerve palsy may require more extensive surgery to achieve satisfactory cosmesis and reduce epiphora. The 'fil d'Arion' technique of encircling the palpebral aperture with a silicone rod inserted deep to the orbicularis muscle, running behind the medial canthal tendon and attached to the lateral orbital rim, is one technique of providing some degree of closure.

Mechanical

Any lesion of the lower lid sufficiently large to distort its position can produce ectropion — e.g., neurofibroma of the lid (Fig. 1.2.8). Treatment is aimed at excision of the lesion, but it may also be necessary to correct any secondary changes due to stretching of the tissues.

Entropion

Congenital (Fig. 1.2.9)

This rare condition is due to hypertrophy of the orbicularis musculature. It may lead to recurrent conjunctivitis. The entropion usually resolves spontaneously, and therefore can be managed using temporary measures such as taping of the lids or everting sutures. Severe cases not amenable to such treatment require excision of an ellipse of skin and orbicularis. Slight overcorrection should be sought.

Involutional (Fig. 1.2.10)

Entropion of the lower lid is most commonly involutional, secondary to laxity of the lid musculature, tendons and tarsal plate. Management is surgical and may involve horizontal shortening of the lid, the creation of a fibrous scar horizontally across the lid to prevent the orbicularis lower in the lid from rolling the lid inwards, or plication of flaccid retractors of the lid. Everting sutures can be used either alone (Quickert–Rathbun suture) as a temporary bedside cure, or in conjunction with the creation of a horizontal scar tissue barrier (the Wies procedure Fig. 1.2.11).

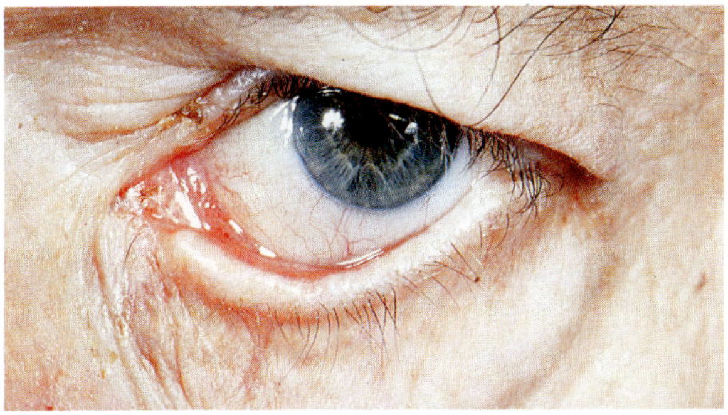

Fig. 1.2.6 Paralytic ectropion in seventh-nerve palsy.

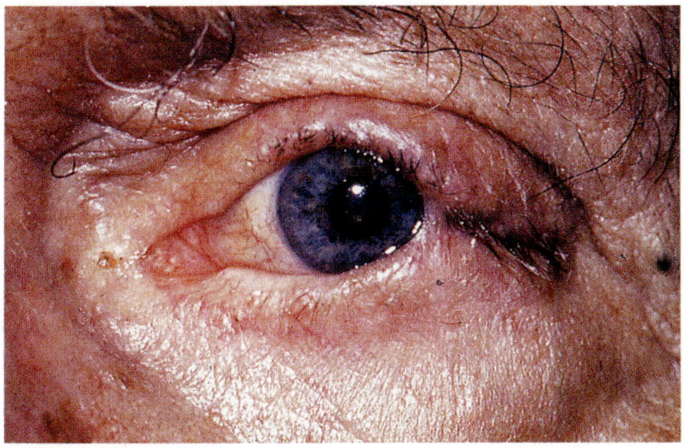

Fig. 1.2.7 Temporary lateral tarsorrhaphy.

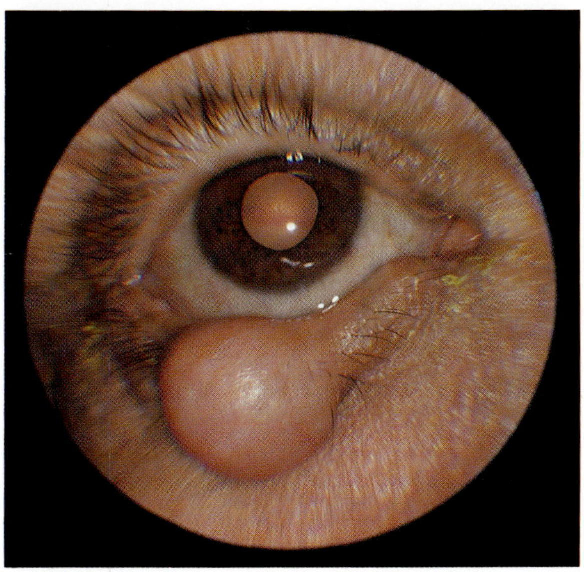

Fig. 1.2.8 Mechanical ectropion due to lower lid neurofibroma.

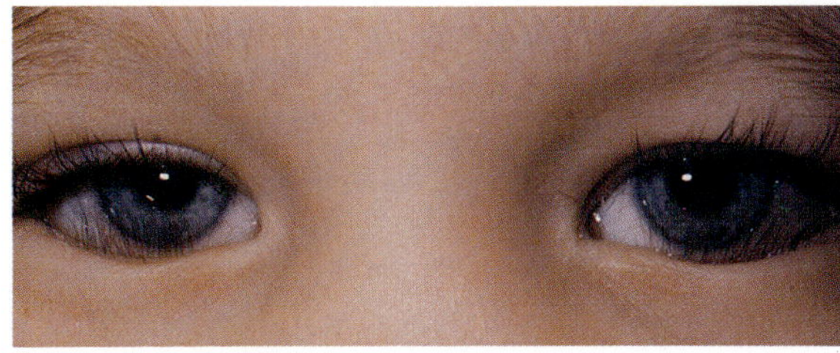

Fig. 1.2.9 Congenital entropion.

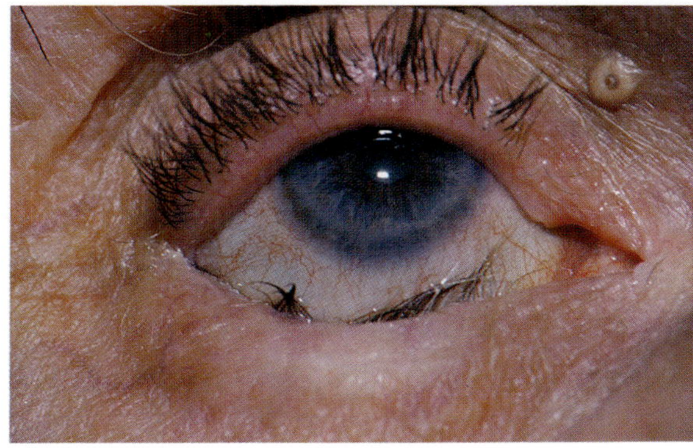

Fig. 1.2.10 Involutional entropion.

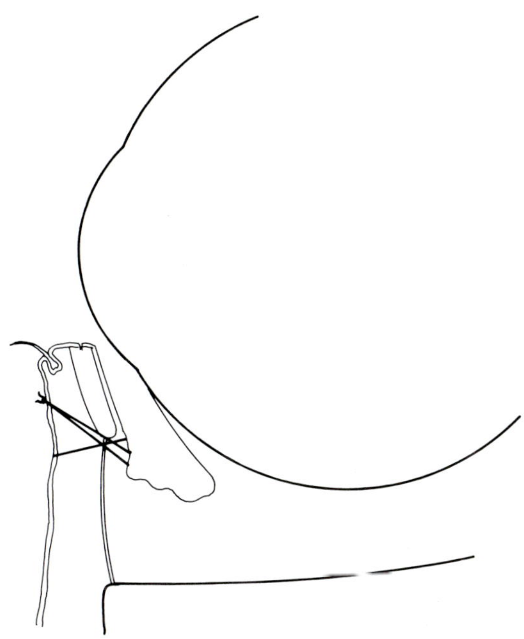

Fig. 1.2.11 The Wies correction of involutional entropion.

Cicatricial (Fig. 1.2.12)

Scarring of the conjunctiva leads to inversion of the lid. Causes include trauma, alkali burns, chronic infection, the Stevens–Johnson syndrome, mucous membrane pemphigoid and chronic allergic disease. Treatment depends on the extent of the scarring: a lid-everting procedure may suffice, often involving tarsal fracture. Mild cases in which the upper tarsal plate is healthy can be managed by rotation of the lid margin only. More severe cicatrization requires lengthening of the shortened posterior lamella by inlay of sclera or nasal cartilage. Such spacers should be covered with mucosa. Associated lid retraction may require release of the levator complex, or lower lid retractors. Surgical measures should be undertaken in conjunction with medical management of any predisposing factors.

Ptosis

Congenital

Congenital ptosis may occur as an isolated condition or in association with an ocular motility defect, such as double elevator palsy, in which reduced activity of the superior rectus and interior oblique muscles is seen (Fig. 1.2.13). Some patients with congenital ptosis exhibit the Marcus–Gunn jaw-winking phenomenon, when the lid moves with mastication or sucking (Fig. 1.2.14 a and b). This generally becomes less noticeable as the child grows. Unilateral congenital ptosis requires early treatment if the visual axis is covered by the lid because of the risk of amblyopia. If there is good levator function, success can be achieved with resection of a segment of this muscle or its aponeurosis, but often dystrophy of the levator necessitates a brow suspension procedure. This involves connection of the upper lid to the frontalis musculature, using either strips of autogenous fascia lata, stored allograft fascia, or non-absorbable macromesh materials.

The blepharophimosis syndrome (Fig. 1.2.15) is inherited in an autosomal dominant manner and consists of bilateral ptosis together with a narrowed palpebral aperture, an inverted medial canthal skin fold, widely spaced canthi and anteversion of the ears. It is variable in severity.

Neurogenic

Third-nerve palsy causes ptosis in association with exotropia, slight intorsion and hypotropia of the eye (Fig. 1.2.16). If the palsy is complete the pupil is also dilated. Treatment should be directed firstly toward correction of the strabismus, followed by surgery to the ptosis. Bell's phenomenon may be reduced, and in such cases care must be taken not to create corneal exposure when lifting the lid. Aberrant regeneration of the third nerve following damage to it may lead to unusual phenomena such as elevation of the lid on adduction of the globe. Horner's syndrome (Fig. 1.2.17) causes a lesser degree of ptosis, with a miosed rather than dilated pupil. Resection of a segment of tarso-conjunctiva (Fasanella–Servat operation) corrects this well in most instances.

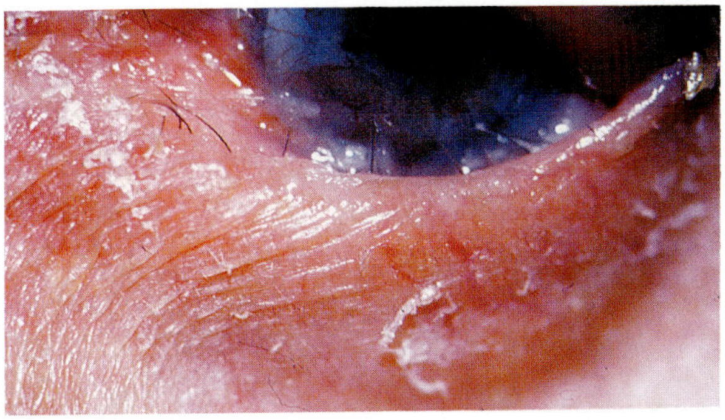

Fig. 1.2.12 Cicatricial entropion.

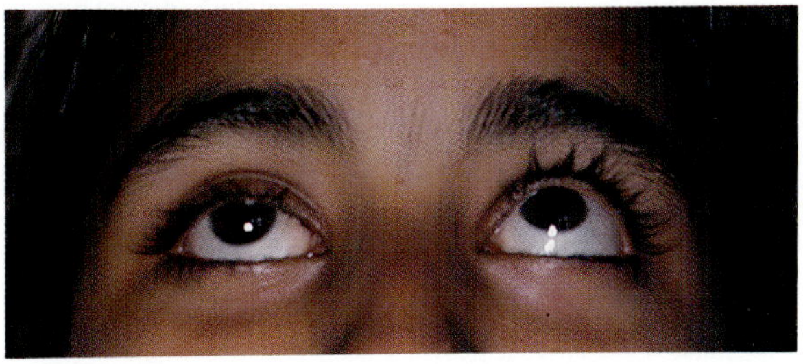

Fig. 1.2.13 Ptosis associated with double elevator palsy of the right eye.

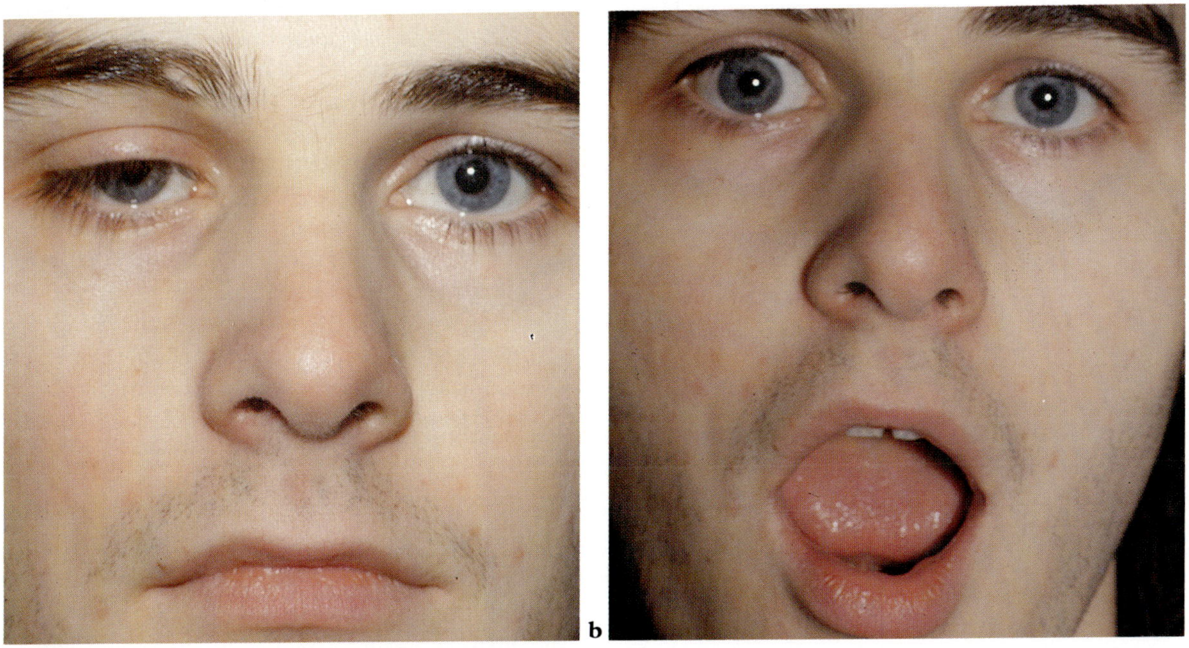

a **b**

Fig. 1.2.14 (a and b) The Marcus–Gunn jaw-winking phenomenon demonstrating reversal of ptosis on mastication.

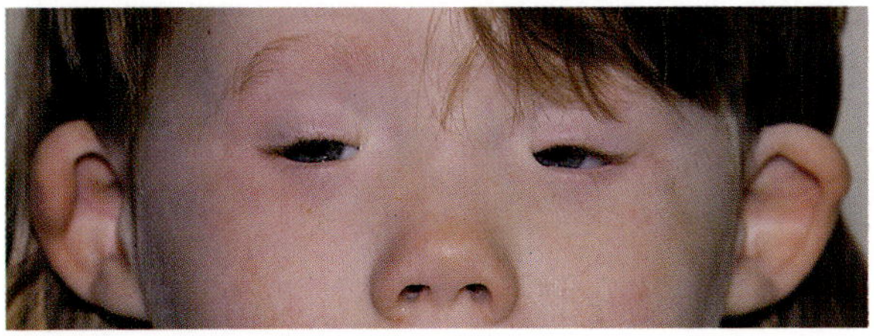

Fig. 1.2.15 The blepharophimosis syndrome (courtesy of Mr J. R. O. Collin).

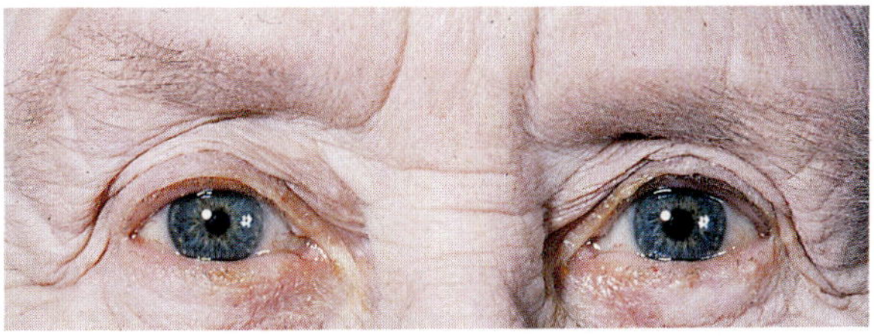

Fig. 1.2.17 Horner's syndrome involving the right eye.

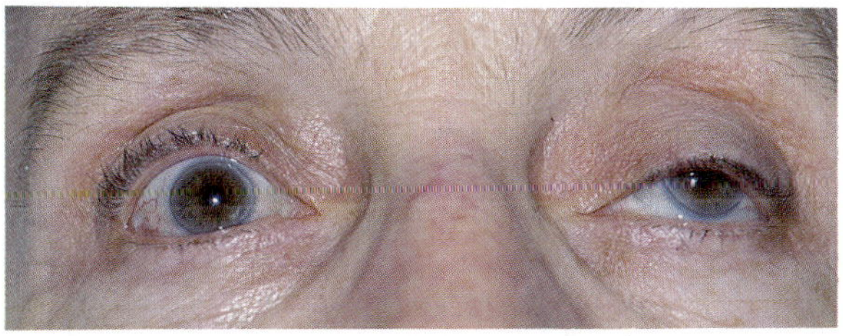

Fig. 1.2.16 Ptosis due to a left-sided third-nerve palsy.

Mechanical

Mechanical ptosis may be caused by any lesion of the upper lid sufficiently large to overcome the retractor musculature (Fig. 1.2.18). Treatment should be directed towards removal of the lesion, but changes which develop secondarily to chronic traction of the tissues may necessitate surgery to the levator complex.

Involutional

Involutional ptosis occurs as a result of loss of tone of the retractors, and laxity of the aponeurosis of the levator palpebrae superioris. If the aponeurosis tears or disinserts from the lid, the skin crease becomes elevated (Fig. 1.2.19). The degree of ptosis and levator function determine the surgical approach, which either involves repair of an aponeurotic defect or resection of levator musculature.

Myogenic

The ocular myopathies include myasthenia gravis, dystrophia myotonica and progressive external ophthalmoplegia; they may all present with ptosis.

Myasthenia gravis causes generalized muscle weakness, particularly towards the end of the day and after exercise, although such fatigue is not always present. The condition is progressive but may present initially with ptosis or extraocular muscle weakness (ocular myasthenia). The diagnosis should be considered in all cases of senile ptosis. Reversal of the ptosis on injection of 10 mg edrophonium (tensilon) is diagnostic. Anticholinesterases can then be used to control the symptoms, although isolated ocular myasthenia often responds better to systemic steroids.

Dystrophia myotonica is a muscular dystrophy which can affect the extraocular muscles and levator complex, and so cause restricted eye movements and ptosis. It may also be associated with characteristic cataract and non-specific corneal changes.

Progressive external ophthalmoplegia is a mitochondrial cytopathy in which there is an increasing limitation of eye movements, usually associated with progressive ptosis, which is the first sign of the disease (Fig. 1.2.20). The condition is associated with a number of neurological abnormalities which include pharyngeal paresis, cerebellar ataxia, spasticity, peripheral neuropathy and cardiac conduction defects. A pigmentary retinopathy may coexist.

Lash malposition

Trichiasis

Lashes may become misdirected by any disease which leads to distortion of the lid margin contour or position, e.g., chronic blepharitis, trachoma, mucous membrane pemphigoid (Fig. 1.2.21). When trichiasis is limited to only a few aberrant lashes, electrolysis of the lash follicles is normally sufficient. More extensive disease should be treated with cryotherapy. A double freeze–thaw cycle to –20°C should be used, with a thermocouple inserted into the lash follicle to monitor the temperature. The ablation of upper lid lashes, in particular, may be cosmetically unsatisfactory, and the associated skin depigmentation may be especially noticeable in dark-skinned individuals. Patients should be warned of these effects.

Distichiasis (Fig. 1.2.22)

Distichiasis is a congenital secondary row of lashes, which arises from the meibomian gland orifices. If the cornea is abraded, cryotherapy of the posterior lamella of the lid following split at the grey line is indicated. In the upper lid, this should be combined with advancement of the posterior lamella in order to prevent the development of entropion.

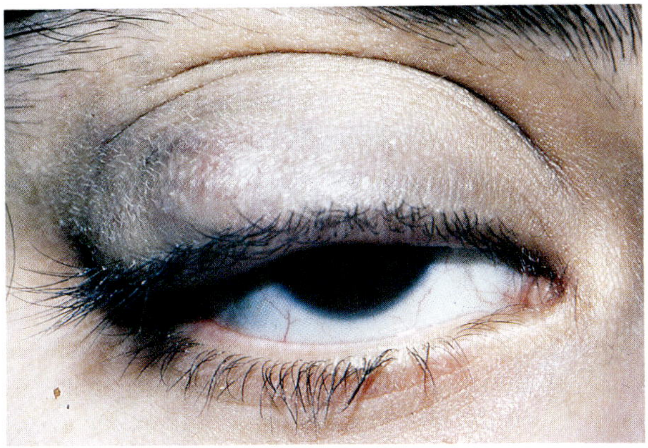

Fig. 1.2.18 Mechanical ptosis due to an upper lid haemangioma.

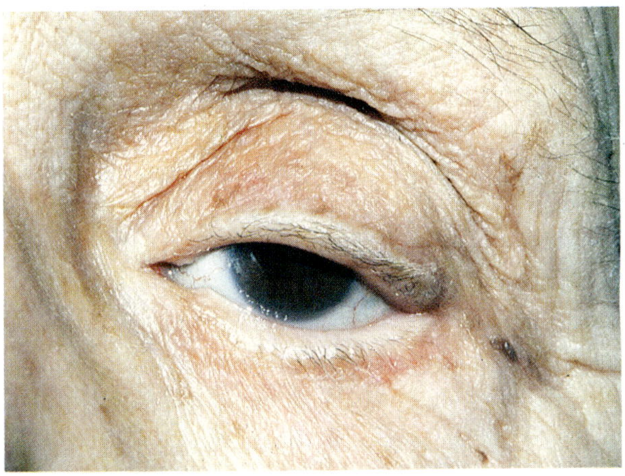

Fig. 1.2.19 Ptosis due to disinsertion of the levator aponeurosis.

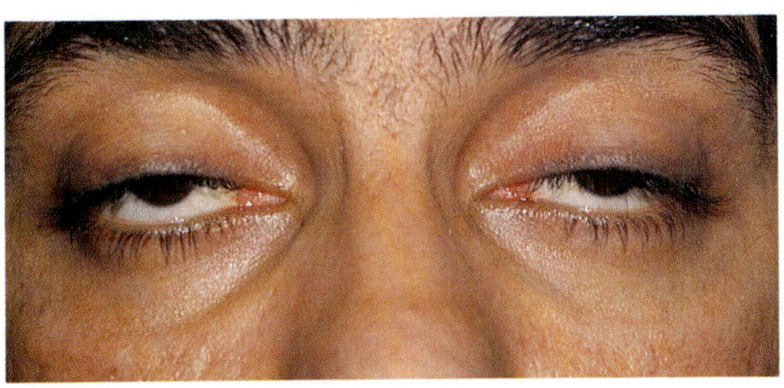

Fig. 1.2.20 Bilateral ptosis in progressive external ophthalmoplegia.

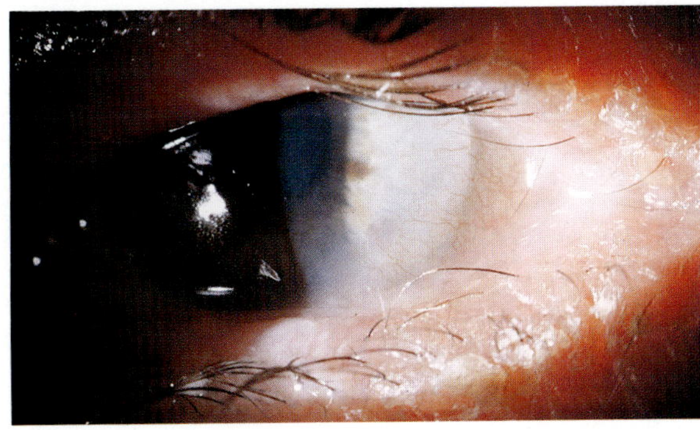

Fig. 1.2.21 Trichiasis caused by mucous membrane pemphigoid.

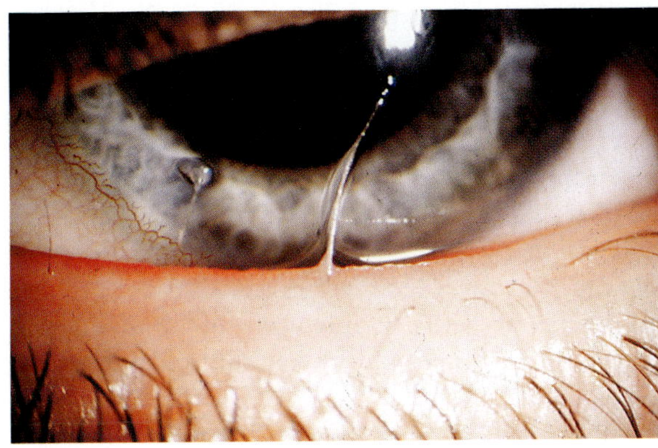

Fig. 1.2.22 Distichiasis. (Courtesy of Mr G. E. Rose)

BENIGN AND INFLAMMATORY LESIONS OF THE EYELIDS

Stye (Fig. 1.3.1)

The stye or hordeolum externum is an acute suppurative staphylococcal infection of a lash follicle and its associated glands. Resolution is usually spontaneous, although removal of the affected lash may aid drainage. Surgical incision is rarely necessary.

Chalazion (Fig. 1.3.2)

This is a granulomatous swelling in the lid, caused by the phagocytosis of retained meibomian gland secretions. Chalazia generally resolve spontaneously, but may persist as firm swellings which require curettage. Alternatively, local injection of triamcinolone has been used to achieve resolution. Recurrent chalazia occur in association with seborrhoeic blepharitis and rosacea. Rarely, adenocarcinoma of the meibomian glands presents in this way, and if suspected the whole lesion should be excised and examined histologically.

Cyst of Zeiss and Moll (Fig. 1.3.3)

These appear as round swellings in the anterior lamella of the lid margin. They require no treatment, but can be excised for cosmetic reasons. Cysts of Zeiss (arrow) are full of sebaceous material and hence are yellow, whereas cysts of Moll contain clear fluid.

Seborrhoeic keratosis (Fig. 1.3.4)

This is also termed seborrhoeic wart or basal cell papilloma. It is a common lesion on exposed skin, which is not premalignant. It appears as a clearly demarcated brownish elevation, which often has a roughened surface, and is sometimes papillary. The degree of pigmentation is variable.

Histologically, the lesion demonstrates hyperkeratosis and an increased thickness of the prickle cell layer. Excision is required only if the diagnosis is in question, or for cosmesis.

Papilloma of lid skin (Fig. 1.3.5)

These benign skin tags with a vascular pedicle require removal only for cosmetic reasons. They are commonly of viral origin.

Xanthelasma (Fig. 1.3.6)

These plaques of lipid in the skin are common in old age, but may also be a manifestation of hyperlipoproteinaemia, often in association with corneal arcus. They can be removed if unsightly, or sufficiently large to cause ptosis, either surgically or by application of trichloracetic acid. When present in those aged less than 45, fasting plasma lipoproteins should be measured in order to detect serious conditions such as familial hypercholesterolaemia which require treatment.

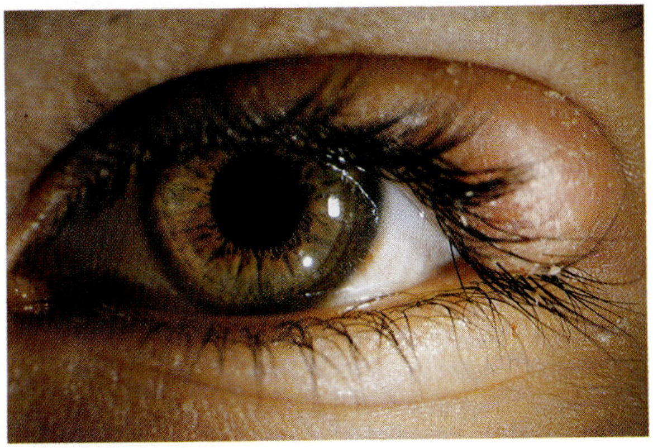

Fig. 1.3.1 Stye (external hordeolum).

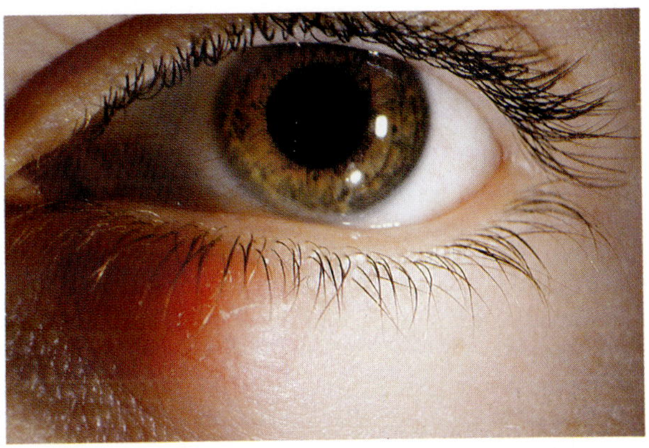

Fig. 1.3.2 Chalazion.

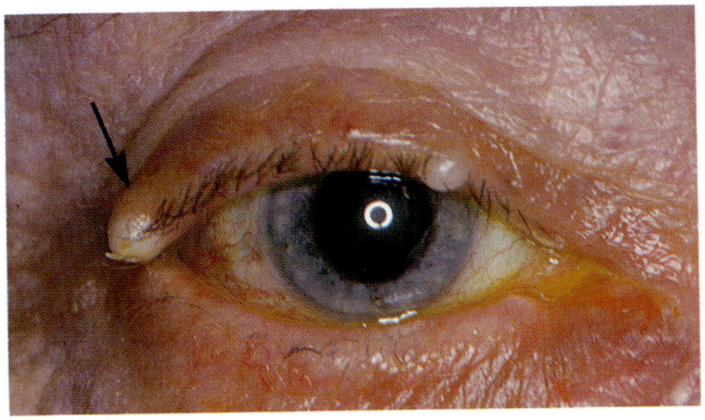

Fig. 1.3.3 Cysts of Zeiss (arrow) and Moll.

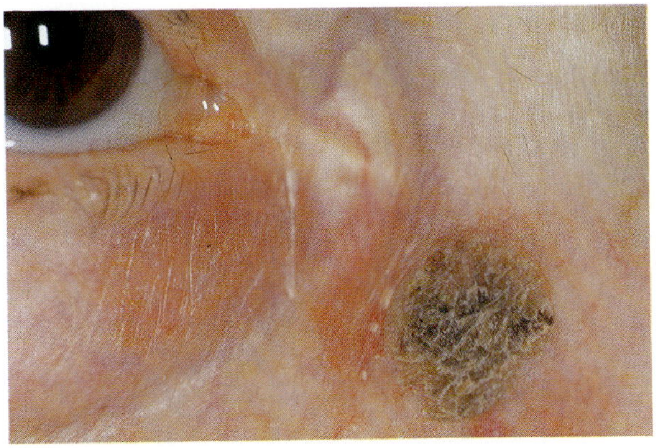

Fig. 1.3.4 Seborrhoeic keratosis of skin in periorbital region.

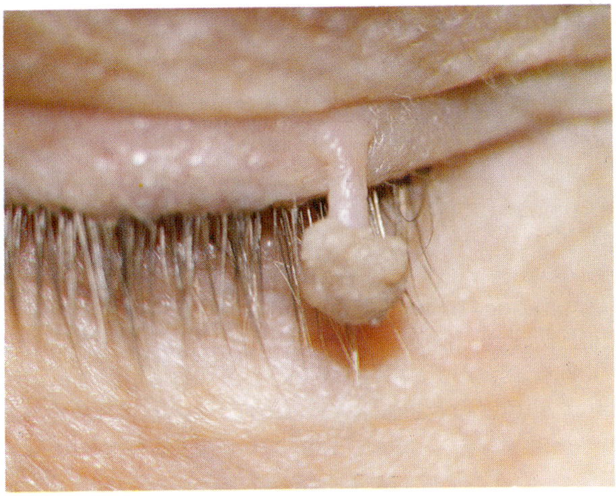

Fig. 1.3.5 Papilloma of upper eyelid.

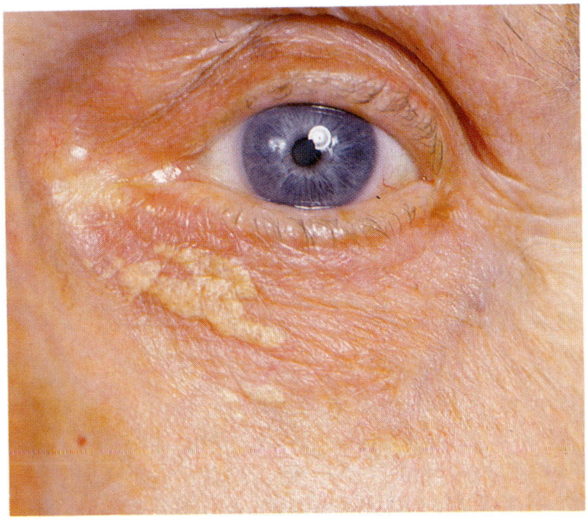

Fig. 1.3.6 Xanthelasma.

Molluscum contagiosum (Fig. 1.3.7)

This is caused by a poxvirus. It is most commonly seen in children, and appears as one or more dome-shaped nodules situated on the lid, with a caseous material in the centre. If situated on the lid margin, the release of viral particles into the conjunctival fornices may provoke a follicular keratoconjunctivitis, often resulting in pannus formation. Treatment requires expression of the lesion after incision, and/or cautery. Cryotherapy has also been used.

Histology is characteristic, demonstrating a lobulated structure with a central crater full of inclusion bodies (Fig. 1.3.8).

Neurofibroma

Neurofibromatosis (von Recklinghausen's disease) is an autosomal dominant disorder which has a number of ocular manifestations. These include lid lesions (Fig. 1.3.9) which can lead to a variety of malpositions. Their identification may be assisted by, or draw attention to, café-au-lait patches of skin pigmentation or multiple cutaneous neurofibromata (Fig. 1.3.10). These latter can rarely become malignant. Neurofibromata of the lid may exist in isolation, without any other evidence of the disease. Upper lid involvement is often associated with glaucoma.

Sturge–Weber syndrome (Fig. 1.3.11)

This syndrome, manifest by the presence of a cutaneous angioma over the distribution of the first and often second divisions of the trigeminal nerve, may be associated with intracranial angiomas, and consequent epilepsy and mental retardation. Associated ipsilateral glaucoma is often refractory to treatment. Ipsilateral choroidal haemangiomas often coexist, and may be extensive.

Haemangioma (Fig. 1.3.12)

Haemangiomas of the lids may occur as isolated lesions presenting at birth or within the first months of life. Although they regress spontaneously, treatment is required if the lid occludes the visual axis, or if the tumour leads to astigmatism, in order to prevent amblyopia. Injection of a combination of triamcinolone and dexamethasone around the tumour base achieves shrinkage of the lesions, and surgery is rarely required.

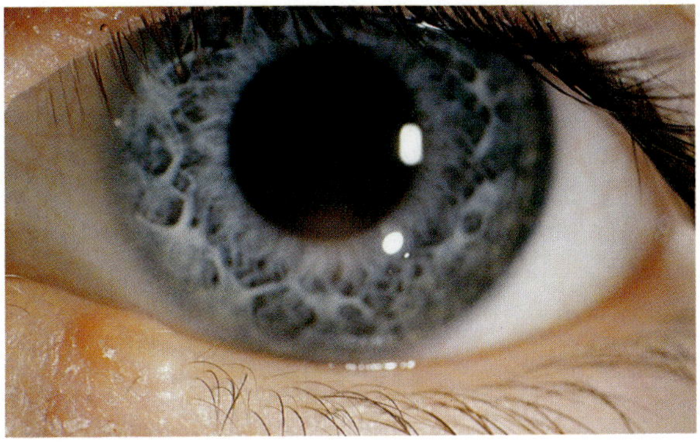

Fig. 1.3.7 Molluscum contagiosum.

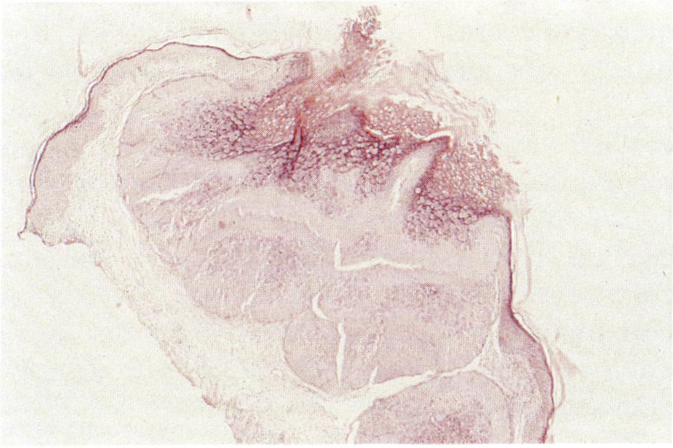

Fig. 1.3.8 Histological section of molluscum contagiosum (haematoxylin and eosin stain).

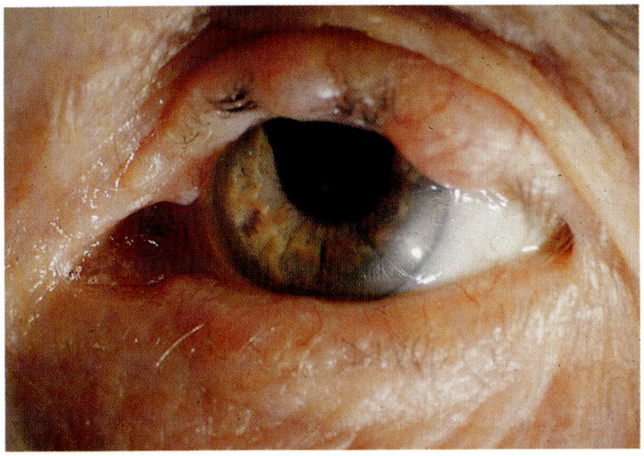

Fig. 1.3.9 Neurofibroma of upper lid.

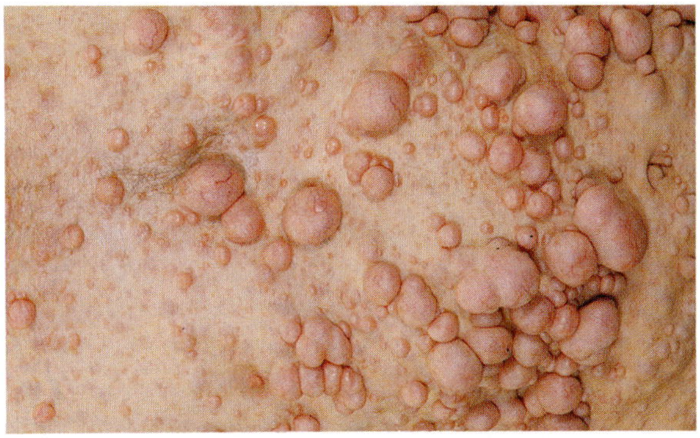

Fig. 1.3.10 Cutaneous neurofibromata in von Recklinghausen's disease.

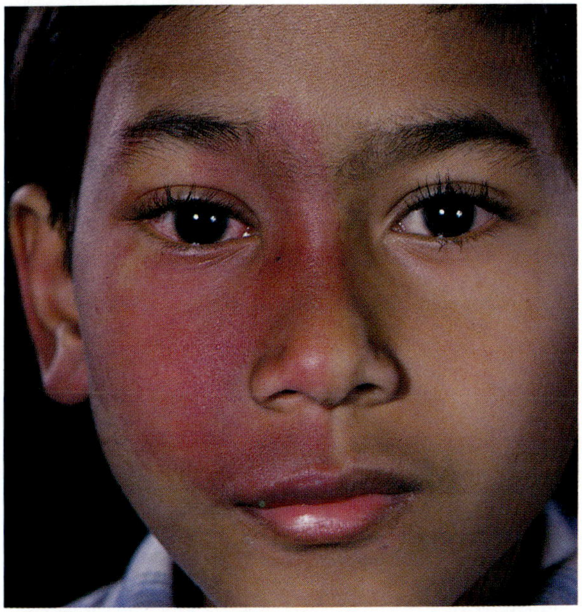

Fig. 1.3.11 The Sturge–Weber syndrome (courtesy of Mr I. G. Rennie).

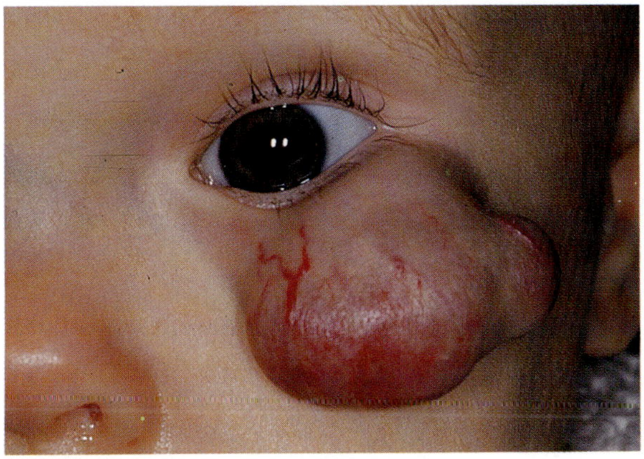

Fig. 1.3.12 Lid haemangioma.

PRE-MALIGNANT AND MALIGNANT LESIONS

Naevus (Fig. 1.4.1)

Benign naevi of the lids and lid margins are common and require no treatment except for cosmetic reasons. Change in size or colour, or onset of bleeding or irritation from a naevus, however, necessitate biopsy of the lesion. Histologically, naevi consist of collections of cells derived from melanocytes. In junctional naevi these are found at the epidermis/dermis interface alone, whereas in compound naevi they are seen also in the dermis. Some deep naevi are purely intradermal.

'Junctional activity' refers to the proliferation of cells at the epidermis/dermis interface, with migration from the epidermis into the dermis. Although normal in early life, such junctional activity after puberty is suggestive of malignancy.

Oculodermal melanocytosis (naevus of Ota) (Fig. 1.4.2)

This condition, which rarely progresses to malignancy, is characterized by pigmentation of the lid skin and adjacent ocular structures (episclera, sclera and uvea). It is often congenital or develops at an early age, and represents a developmental disorder of the neural crest. The pigmentation may increase with age, both in extent and intensity. An increased incidence of glaucoma is associated with the condition, due to abnormal development of the iridocorneal angle.

Solar keratosis (Fig. 1.4.3)

This is also termed senile keratosis, actinic keratosis, or squamous cell carcinoma grade a half. These terms reflect the frequent occurrence in the elderly, increased incidence following exposure to sunlight, and malignant potential of the lesion. The appearance may be of a cutaneous horn or of scaly plaques. This latter change reflects lack of cohesion between cells. Because of their malignant potential, the lesions should be excised.

Intraepithelial carcinoma (Bowen's disease) (Fig. 1.4.4)

This form of carcinoma-in-situ, which tends to progress to squamous cell carcinoma, is rare on the eyelids, and is usually located on non-exposed parts of the body. Its appearance of discrete red plaques mimics psoriasis and the diagnosis is often not made until infiltrative carcinoma has supervened.

Xeroderma pigmentosum (Fig. 1.4.5)

This is an autosomal recessive disorder of DNA repair which leads to a progressive involvement of exposed areas by epithelial neoplasms. It is usually first manifest in early childhood by the presence of numerous freckles with surrounding erythema and later progresses to the development of multiple telangiectases. A variety of tumours, which include basal cell carcinoma, squamous cell carcinoma, malignant melanoma and sarcoma, develop subsequently. Both the eyelids and conjunctiva may be involved. The disease is often relentlessly progressive leading to an early demise.

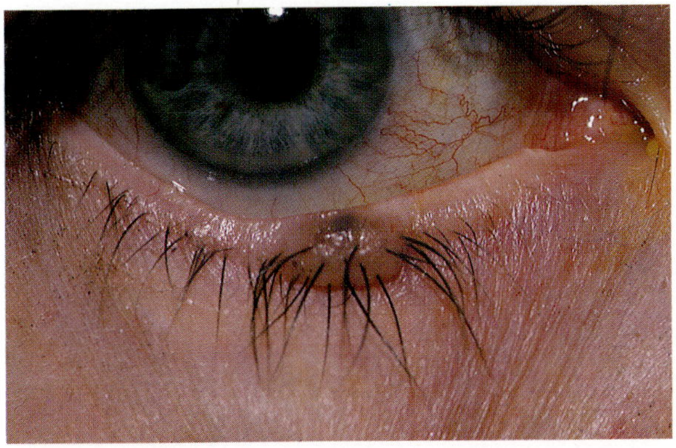

Fig. 1.4.1 Benign naevus of the lower lid.

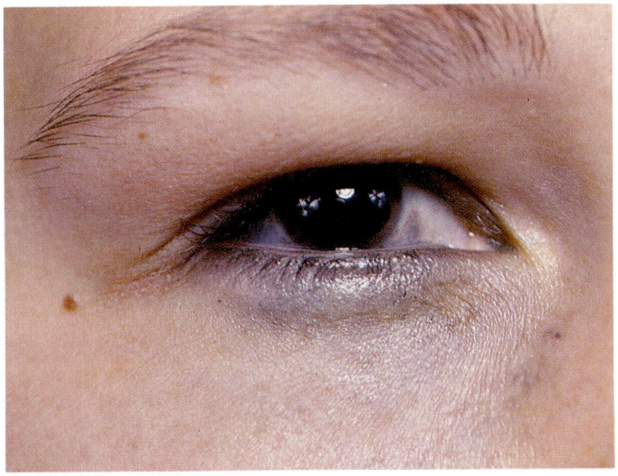

Fig. 1.4.2 Oculodermal melanocytosis (naevus of Ota).

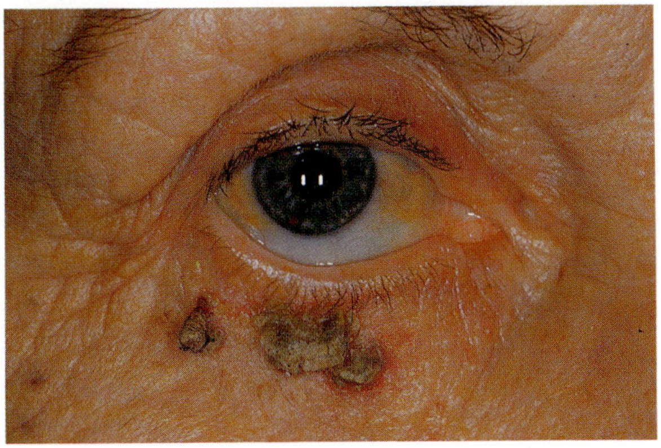

Fig. 1.4.3 Solar keratosis.

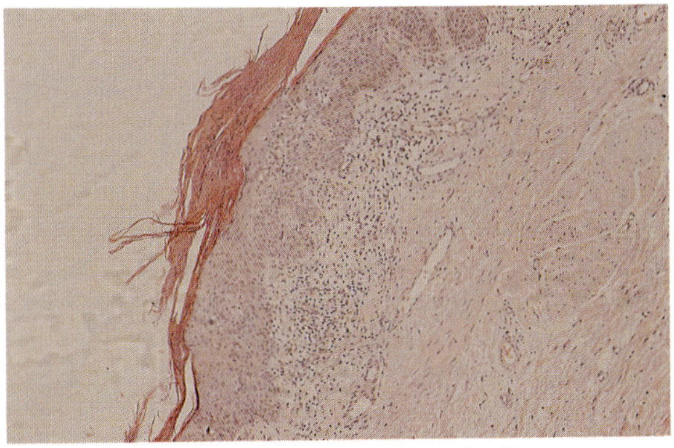

Fig. 1.4.4 Histological section of Bowen's disease (haematoxylin and eosin stain) demonstrating epidermal hyperplasia (courtesy of the Department of Dermatology, Royal Hallamshire Hospital).

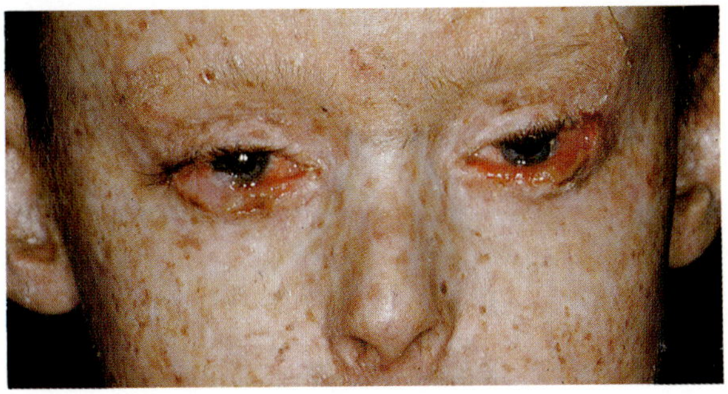

Fig. 1.4.5 Xeroderma pigmentosum (courtesy of Mr M. J. Potts).

Keratoacanthoma

This appears in the elderly and undergoes spontaneous remission after a phase of rapid growth. The appearance is of an ulcer filled with a keratin plug (Fig. 1.4.6) which is discharged as the lesion begins to heal. Failure of resolution within six months should arouse suspicion of malignancy. Histology can be confusing, however, and the lesion can be mistaken for squamous cell carcinoma if it is biopsied during the phase of active growth (Fig. 1.4.7).

Basal cell carcinoma

This is a common tumour of the lids and face, particularly in the elderly and following chronic exposure to sunlight. It almost never metastasizes, but complete surgical removal is necessary to prevent local extension and recurrence. The most common appearance is of a nodular tumour (Fig. 1.4.8), but ulcerative or cicatrizing lesions (Fig. 1.4.9) may occur as well as more diffuse (morphoeic) tumours. Determination of the limits of extension of this latter type in particular may be difficult. Frozen section control of excision reduces recurrence rate, which, even using this technique, exceeds 10% at five-year follow up. Sequential excisions, based on systematic microscopic scanning of the entire under-surface and edges of each layer of accurately labelled tissue (Mohs' surgery) has reduced recurrence rates.

Repair of the lids following adequate resection may require extensive reconstructive surgery. In cases of repeated recurrences or multiple tumours, or where tissue availability precludes conventional repair, the 'laissez-faire' technique of allowing granulation to close a defect will often achieve a satisfactory functional result, even though cosmesis is compromised (Fig. 1.4.10a and b). Other therapeutic options include cryotherapy or radiotherapy if surgical excision is not possible.

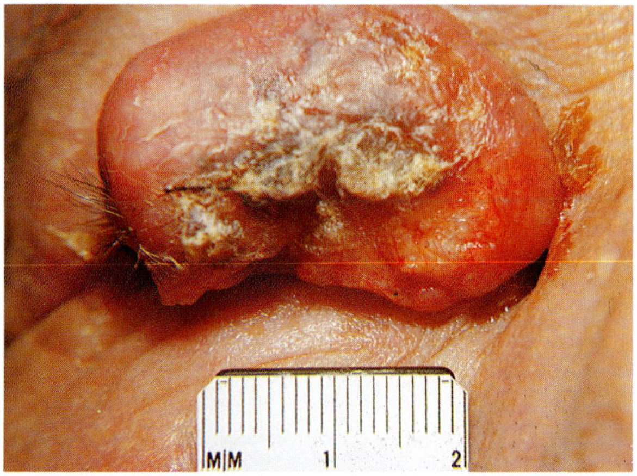

Fig. 1.4.6 Keratoacanthoma.

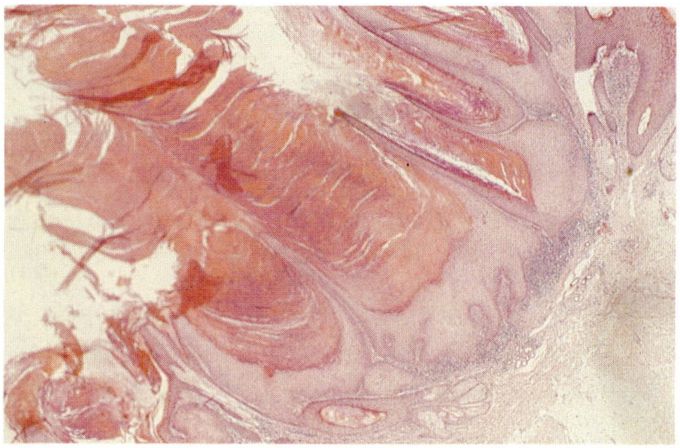

Fig. 1.4.7 Histology of keratoacanthoma demonstrating keratin plug (haematoxylin and eosin stain).

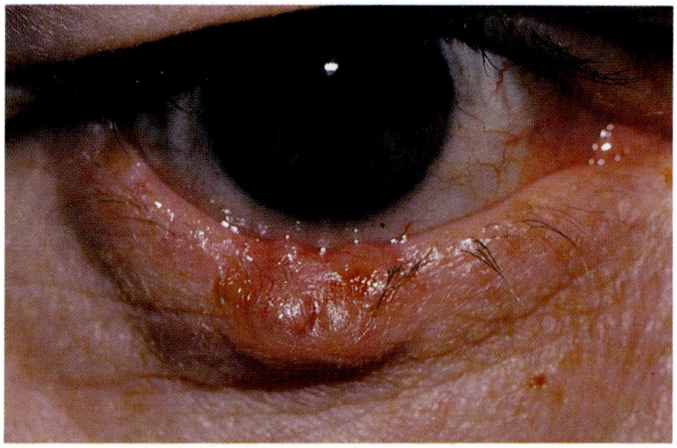

Fig. 1.4.8 Nodular basal cell carcinoma.

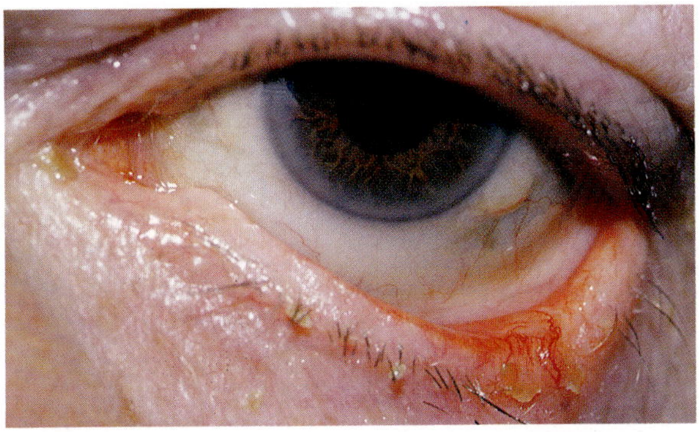

Fig. 1.4.9 Cicatricial basal cell carcinoma leading to ectropion of the lower lid.

a

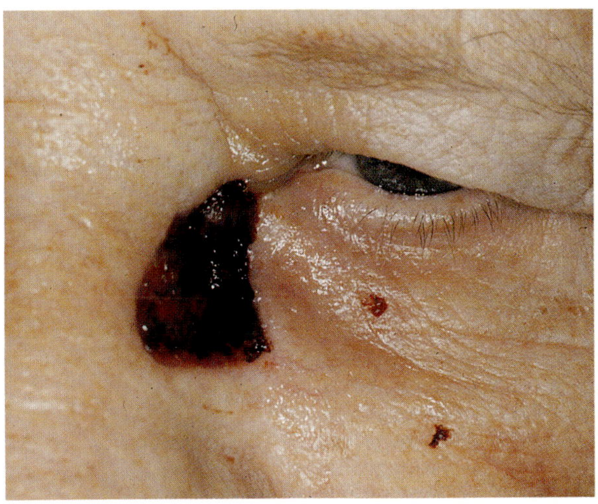

b

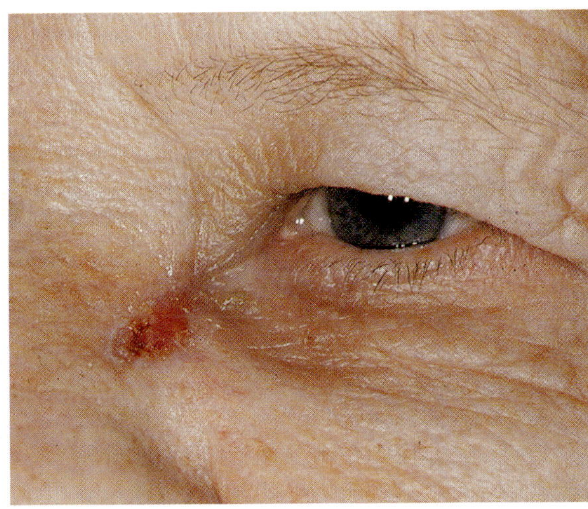

Fig. 1.4.10 A nasally situated basal cell carcinoma (**a**) removed and the wound left to granulate (laissez-faire); (**b**) six weeks later.

A tumour situated nasally (Fig. 1.4.11) may occlude either or both canaliculi directly, or involve them in its excision.

Basal cell carcinomata may be multiple, in particular when found in association with either the naevoid basal cell carcinoma syndrome, or xeroderma pigmentosum. These are hereditary disorders predisposing to cutaneous tumours.

Sebaceous adenocarcinoma (Fig. 1.4.12)

This is a rare tumour, and arises from either the meibomian glands of the tarsal plate, or the glands of Zeiss and Moll. It is notorious for masquerading as chronic unilateral blepharitis, keratoconjunctivitis, or recurrent chalazion. The consequent delay in diagnosis is responsible for the poor prognosis in a significant proportion of cases, and a high index of suspicion should therefore be maintained for this lesion. Any suspicious condition of the conjunctiva or the lid should be biopsied. The specimen should include the full thickness of the lid, and fresh tissue should be examined histologically with fat stains.

The tumour spreads locally, and may infiltrate the orbit, but also metastasizes through the lymphatics and haematogenously. It is most commonly seen in the elderly, but occasionally in the young, especially following irradiation (e.g., for retinoblastoma).

The treatment for isolated lid disease is complete surgical excision with histological control. Pagetoid spread may make identification of the extent of the lesion difficult. If the orbit is involved, in the absence of diffuse metastases, exenteration is indicated. Although the tumour does not respond well to radiotherapy, this may offer useful palliation in extensive disease, or in patients unsuitable for surgery.

Squamous cell carcinoma (Fig. 1.4.13)

This is also a rare tumour, usually being preceded by solar keratosis, or carcinoma in situ. Although basal cell carcinoma is forty times as common on the lids, a lesion in the outer canthal region or upper lid is more likely to be a squamous cell carcinoma. The tumour may present as an indurated ulcer, a nodule, or a papillary growth, and there is usually extensive keratinization. It spreads to the regional lymph nodes, as well as perineurally into the central nervous system, and therefore requires aggressive management by surgical excision and/or radiotherapy.

Melanoma (Fig. 1.4.14)

Malignant melanoma of the lids may arise from a pre-existing skin or conjunctival naevus, or de novo. It is a highly unpredictable tumour, and often disseminates rapidly. Tumours greater than 1.5 mm thick are associated with a particularly poor survival rate, and a nodular histological pattern is also a sinister prognostic indicator. The lesion may be amelanotic, and therefore detected late. Definition of the extent of systemic spread should precede any radical local resection, but management remains controversial.

Kaposi's sarcoma (Fig. 1.4.15)

This rare angiosarcomatous tumour is characteristically found in immunocompromised patients, and in particular in association with the acquired immune deficiency syndrome (AIDS). It appears as a chronic, indolent reddish/purple macule or papule. A number of treatments have been tried, including radiotherapy, single-agent or combination chemotherapy, and the use of α-interferons.

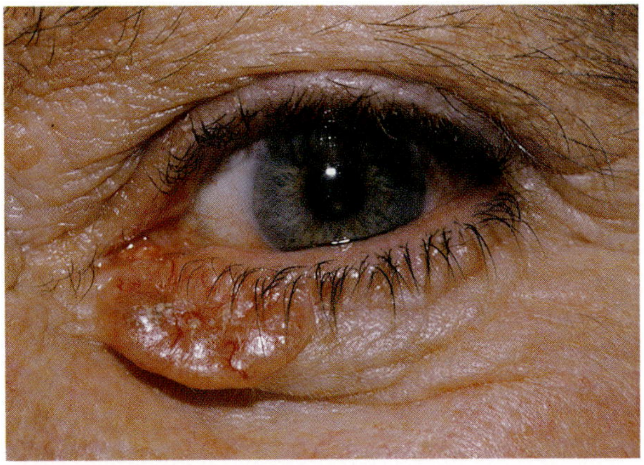

Fig. 1.4.11 Basal cell carcinoma involving the lower canaliculus.

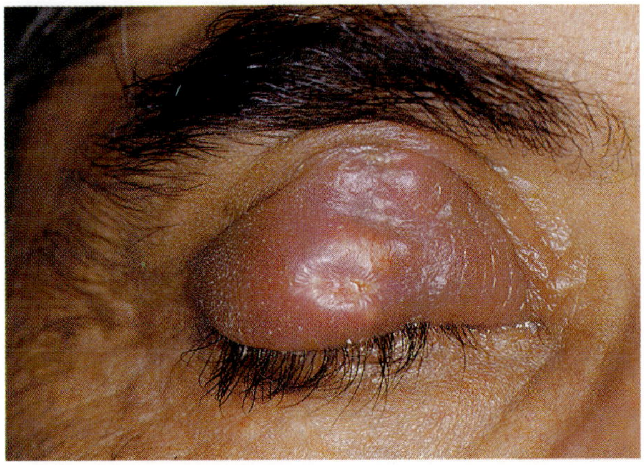

Fig. 1.4.12 Sebaceous adenocarcinoma of the upper eyelid.

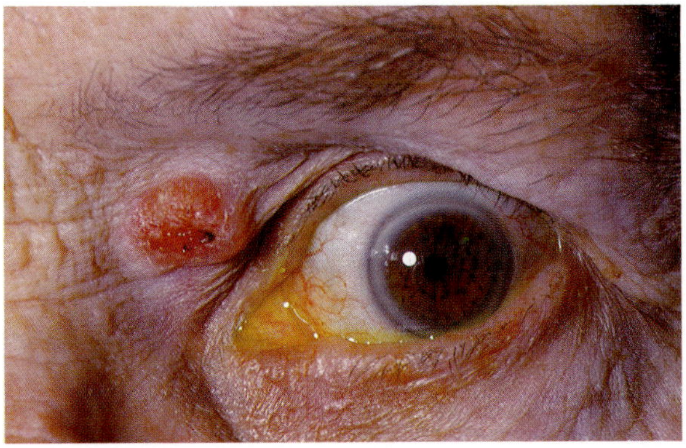

Fig. 1.4.13 Squamous cell carcinoma.

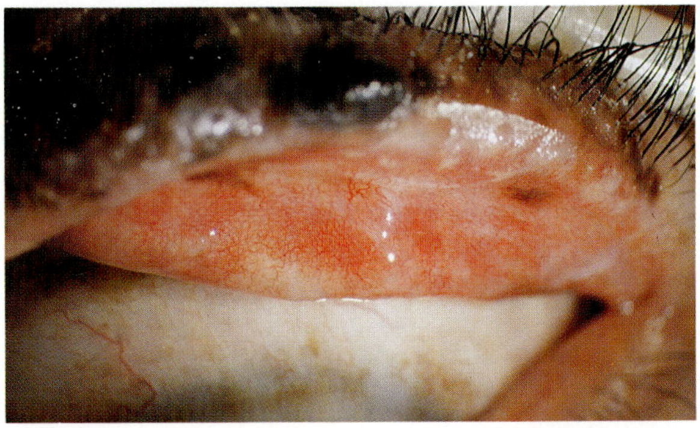

Fig. 1.4.14 Malignant melanoma of the eyelid skin.

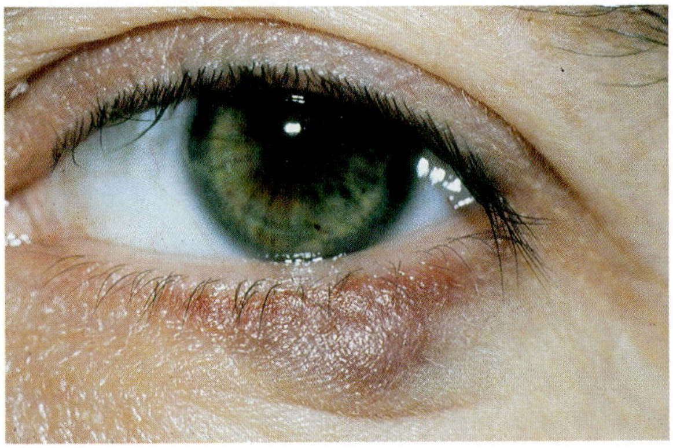

Fig. 1.4.15 Kaposi's sarcoma of the lower eyelid (courtesy of Dr N. P. Smith).

BLEPHARITIS

Blepharitis is an extremely common disorder characterized by symptoms of chronic irritation and foreign body sensation, burning and itching of the eyes and an ocular discharge. It is useful to classify blepharitis into several groups with differing features, associations and complications:

1. staphylococcal
2. seborrhoeic
   - alone
   - mixed seborrhoeic/staphylococcal
   - seborrhoeic with meibomian seborrhoea
   - seborrhoeic with secondary meibomitis
3. primary meibomitis.

(After McCulley et al 1982.)

Staphylococcal (Fig. 1.5.1)

This has a history of recurrent short exacerbations alternating with periods of remission. Foreign body sensation is the predominant symptom, and the eyelids show a characteristic dry, fibrinous scale, often with underlying lid margin ulceration.

The lids are oedematous and inflamed, and the eyelashes may be misdirected (trichiasis) or absent (madarosis) (Fig. 1.5.2).

Frequently, growth of an eyelash causes elevation of the surrounding fibrin scale, forming a collarette (Fig. 1.5.3). The posterior lid margin is normal.

There may be associated chronic papillary conjunctivitis, toxic epithelial keratopathy and keratoconjunctivitis sicca. Local hypersensitivity responses to staphylococcal antigen may occur in the form of marginal keratitis (Fig. 1.5.4) and phlyctenulosis.

Late complications include chronic lid oedema, lid margin malpositions, conjunctival scarring and corneal vascularization.

Whilst *Staphylococcus aureus* can be cultured in some patients, most harbour coagulase-negative staphylococcal species on the lid margin.

Seborrhoeic

Seborrhoeic blepharitis may occur alone or more commonly in association with meibomian gland disease.

The disease course is more chronic with few variations in intensity. A burning sensation is particularly troublesome, and symptoms often far exceed the severity of clinical signs.

Lid scaling is more greasy, and the lids are generally less inflamed (Fig. 1.5.5).

A chronic papillary conjunctivitis is common, but keratoconjunctivitis sicca is seen less frequently than in staphylococcal blepharitis.

Keratitis is unusual unless the meibomian glands are involved.

Mixed staphylococcal/seborrhoeic blepharitis shows features of both, with a similar variation in symptoms with time.

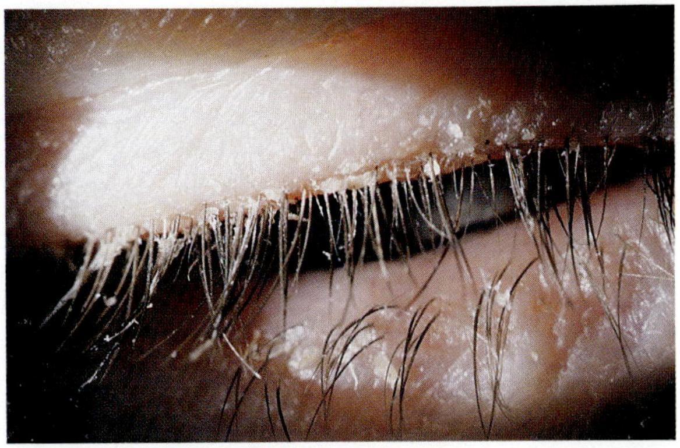

Fig. 1.5.1 Staphylococcal blepharitis.

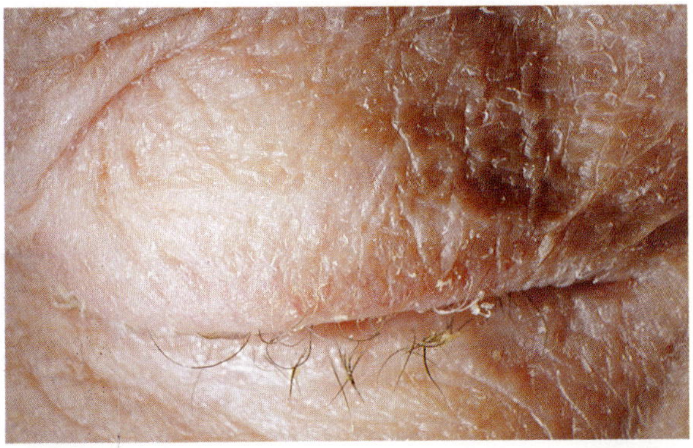

Fig. 1.5.2 Madarosis.

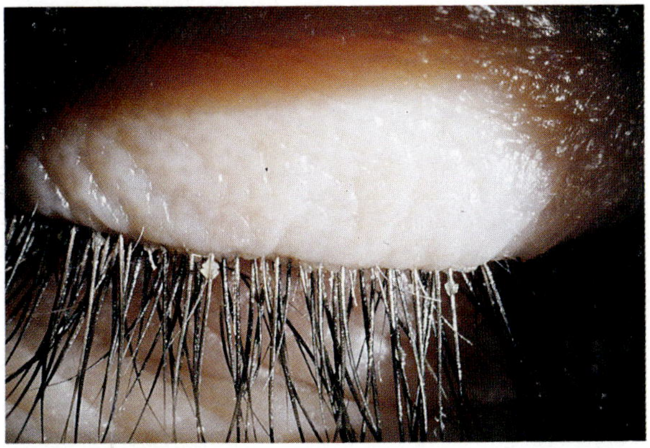

Fig. 1.5.3 Collarettes.

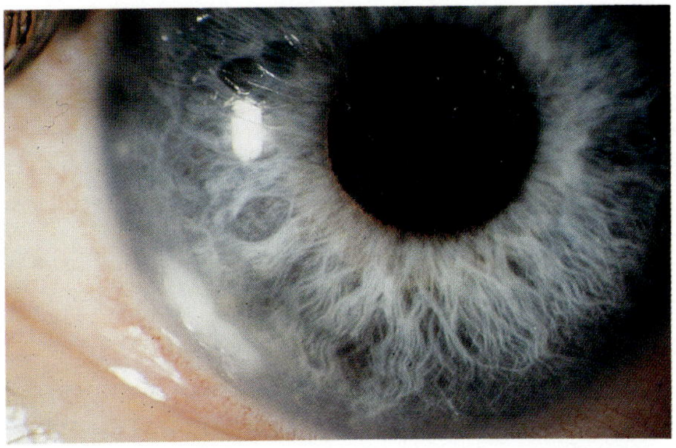

Fig. 1.5.4 Marginal keratitis.

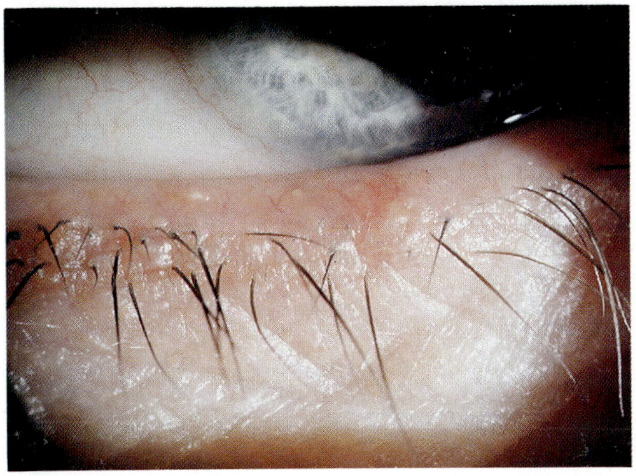

Fig. 1.5.5 Greasy scales in seborrhoeic blepharitis.

Meibomian gland disease in association with seborrhoeic blepharitis is responsible for most of the symptoms and appears as an excess of meibum with dilated glands and a frothy tear film (meibomian seborrhoea, Fig. 1.5.6) or patches of inflamed and occluded glands (secondary meibomitis, Fig. 1.5.7).

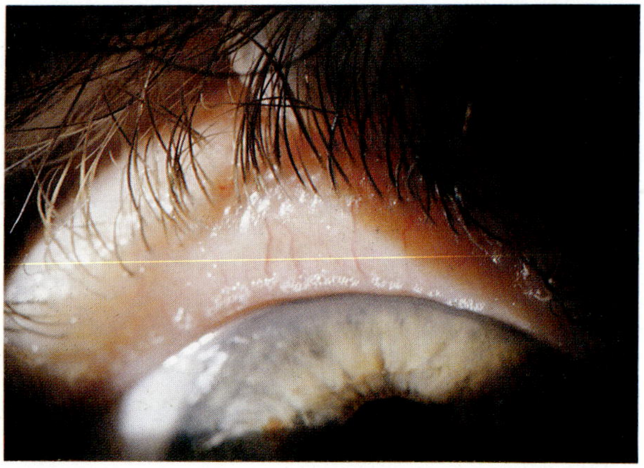

Fig. 1.5.6 Meibomian seborrhoea.

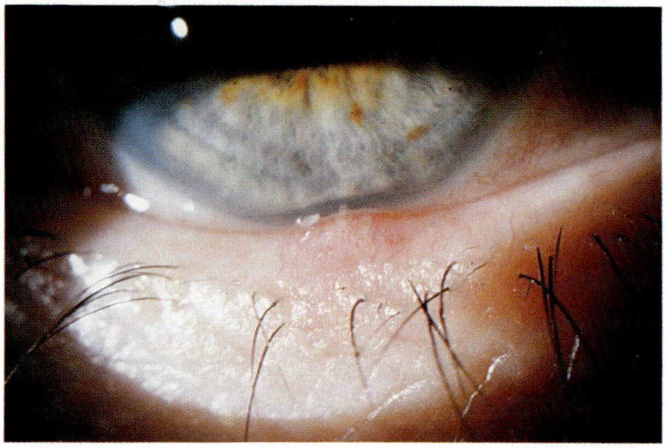

Fig. 1.5.7 Secondary meibomitis.

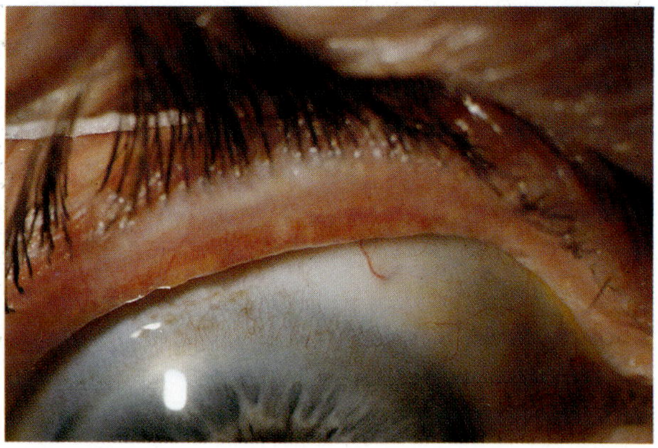

Fig. 1.5.8 Primary meibomitis.

Primary meibomitis (Fig. 1.5.8)

Some patients show involvement of only the posterior lid margin. All the meibomian glands are abnormal, with pouting of their occluded orifices and reduced expressibility of meibum (Fig. 1.5.9). There is a high incidence of punctate keratopathy and papillary conjunctivitis in these patients (meibomian keratoconjunctivitis).

Seborrhoeic dermatitis (Fig. 1.5.10)

This is seen in patients with seborrhoeic blepharitis, both with and without meibomian gland disease, and also in those with primary meibomitis. Greasy scaling is seen predominantly on the scalp and brow, often in association with dandruff.

Demodex (Fig. 1.5.11)

Demodex folliculorum is a mite that is commonly found at the base of the lashes and in the depths of the lash follicle in patients with blepharitis and those with normal lids. Its role in the pathogenesis of blepharitis and other dermatoses such as rosacea is not clear.

Pediculosis (Fig. 1.5.12)

Infestation of the eyelids with lice is a rare cause of blepharitis. It is seen predominantly in children. Treatment consists of a single application of a malathion based lotion.

Rosacea

Rosacea is a common facial dermatosis with erythema, telangiectasis, papules, pustules and sebaceous gland hypertrophy. It is typically found on the forehead, nose, cheeks and chin (Fig. 1.5.13), but the ears, neck and chest can also be affected.

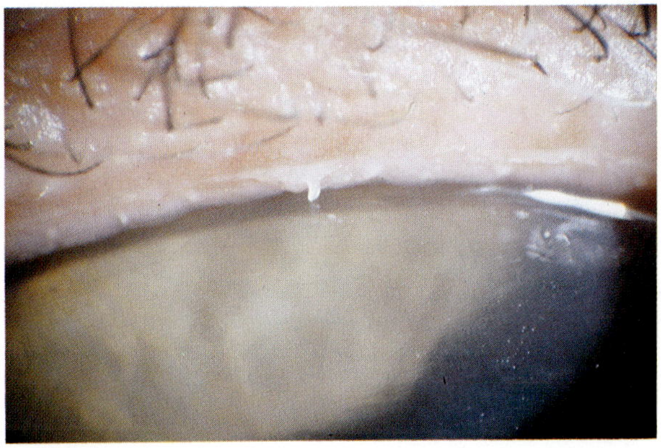

Fig. 1.5.9 Grossly abnormal meibum expressed from gland orifice.

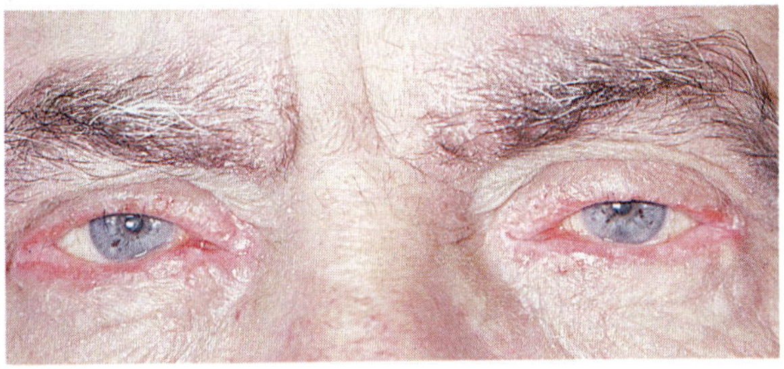

Fig. 1.5.10 Seborrhoeic dermatitis.

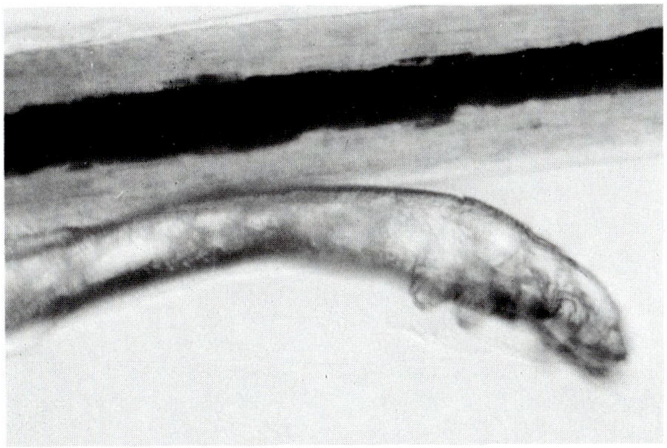

Fig. 1.5.11 *Demodex folliculorum* adjacent to eyelash.

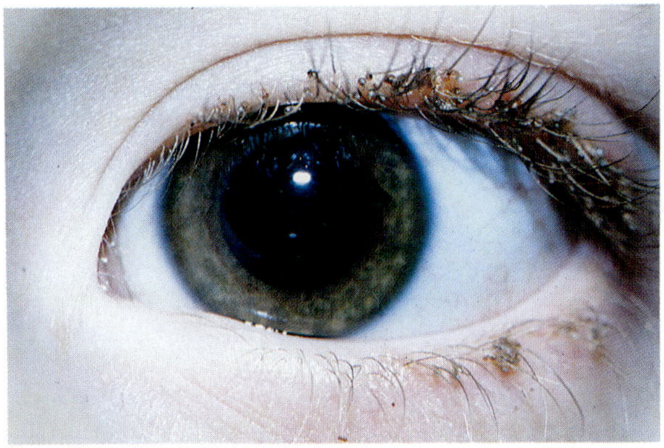

Fig. 1.5.12 Pediculosis.

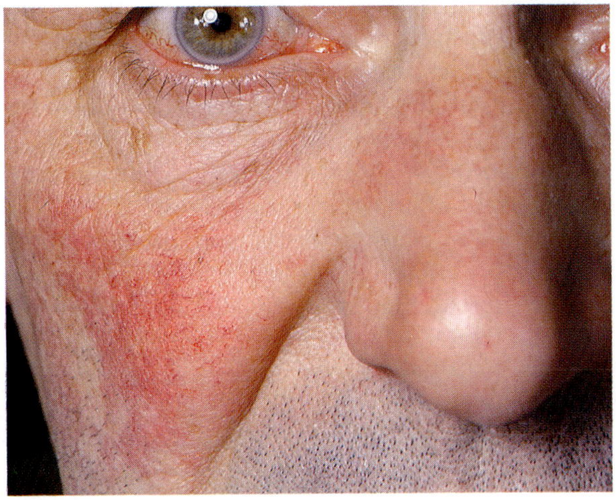

Fig. 1.5.13 Rosacea.

The eye is frequently involved, with lid margin telangiectasia (Fig. 1.5.14), blepharitis, meibomitis, chalazia, conjunctival infection and corneal vascularization, thinning and scarring.

Both skin and ocular manifestations respond to oral antibiotics such as tetracycline, trimethoprim and minocycline, but treatment is often prolonged and relapses are common when it is stopped.

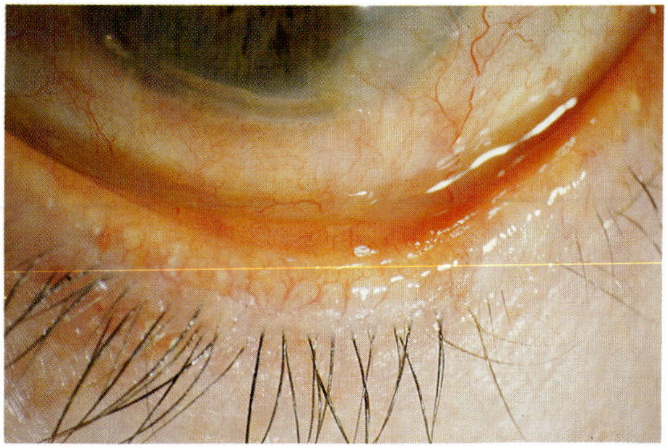

Fig. 1.5.14 Lid margin telangiectasia in acne rosacea.

Management of blepharitis

It is essential to tell the sufferer about the chronicity of the disease, and that treatment will need to be repeated when symptoms recur. The mainstay of treatment is lid hygiene, which the patient must be taught. Several methods are available. The lid margins should be scrubbed with cotton buds dipped in baby shampoo, water or dilute bicarbonate of soda, and then rinsed with water (Fig. 1.5.15). A number of proprietory cleansing solutions are also available.

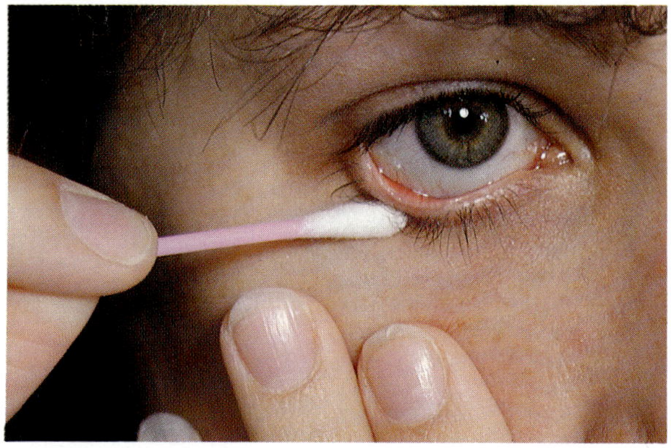

Fig. 1.5.15 Method of lid hygiene.

In addition, some patients respond to a course of topical antibiotics applied to the base of the lashes after lid hygiene.

Since there is a high incidence of keratoconjunctivitis sicca, tear substitutes should be prescribed at least during an acute exacerbation.

Meibomitis and meibomian seborrhoea should also be treated with oral tetracycline (250 mg four times a day for one month, followed by 250 mg once a day for two months). Meibomian gland disease however is often quite resistant to therapy.

FURTHER READING

General

Korting G W 1973 The skin and eye. W B Saunders, Philadelphia

Mackie R M (ed) 1984 Milne's dermatopathology. Arnold, London

McCord C D Jr, Tanenbaum M (eds) 1987 Oculoplastic surgery, 2nd edition. Raven Press, New York

Anatomy

Jakobiec F A, Iwamoto Takeo 1983 Ocular adnexa: introduction to lids, conjunctiva and orbit. In: Duane T D, Jaeger E A (eds) Biochemical foundations of ophthalmology. Harper and Row, Philadelphia

Malpositions

Collin J R O 1989 A manual of systematic eyelid surgery, 2nd edition. Churchill Livingstone, Edinburgh

Levine Mark R 1988 Manual of oculoplastic surgery. Churchill Livingstone, New York

Benign and inflammatory lesions

Deady J P, Willshaw H E 1986 Vascular hamartomas in childhood. Transactions of the Ophthalmological Society of the United Kingdom 105: 712–716

Lucas D R (ed) 1989 Greer's ocular pathology. Blackwell Scientific Publications, Oxford

Pre-malignant and malignant lesions

Dugel P U, Gill P S, Frangieh G T, Rao N A 1990 Ocular adnexal Kaposi's sarcoma in acquired immunodeficiency syndrome. Ophthalmology 110: 500–503

Kass L G, Hornblass A 1989 Sebaceous carcinoma of the ocular adnexa. Survey of Ophthalmology 33: 477–490

Mohs F E 1986 Micrographic surgery for the microscopically controlled excision of eyelid cancer: history and development. Advances in Ophthalmic and Plastic Reconstruction Surgery 5: 381–408

Blepharitis

Browning D J, Proia A D 1986 Ocular rosacea. Survey of Ophthalmology 31: 145–158

McCulley J P, Dougherty J M, Deneau D G 1982 Classification of chronic blepharitis. Ophthalmology 89: 1173–1180

Norn M S 1970 *Demodex folliculorum.* Acta Ophthalmologica Supplementum 108: 1–85

Smolin G, Friedlaender M H (eds) 1987 Management of the dry eye. International Ophthalmology Clinics 27

2
THE CONJUNCTIVA

ANATOMY

The conjunctiva consists of a non-keratinizing stratified columnar epithelium, supported by a vascular substantia propria. Its histology varies with anatomical position.

Bulbar conjunctiva begins at the corneo-scleral limbus, where it is more squamous, and firmly adherent to the globe. On the surface of the globe, and extending out into the fornices, the conjunctiva is loosely adherent and easily distended by fluid.

The forniceal conjunctiva is richly supplied with goblet cells (Fig. 2.1.1), which are mucus-secreting apocrine glands. Mucus coats the conjunctival and corneal surface and acts as a lubricant, protecting and hydrating the epithelia, and also lowers the surface tension of the tear film.

The palpebral conjunctiva (Fig. 2.1.2) begins at the muco-cutaneous junction of the eyelid (Fig. 2.1.3) and is firmly fixed to the underlying tarsal plate.

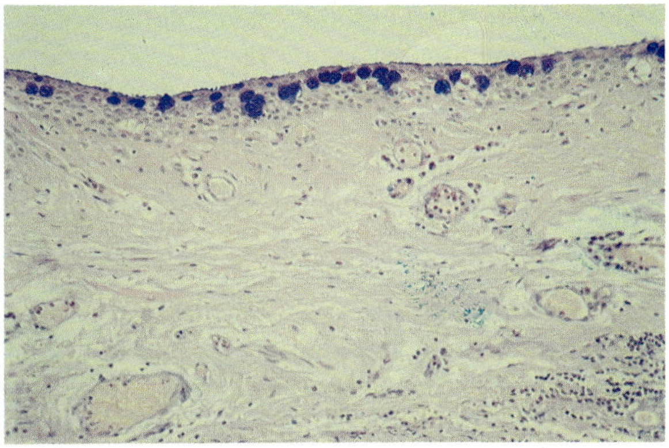

Fig. 2.1.1 Conjunctival goblet cells stained with Alcian Blue.

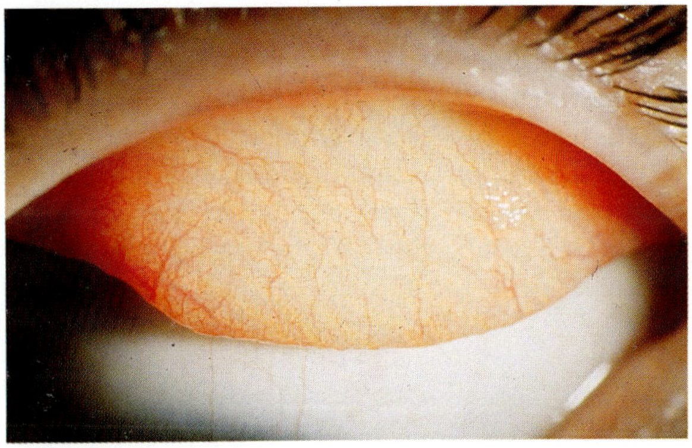

Fig. 2.1.2 The upper lid everted to demonstrate palpebral conjunctiva adherent to the tarsal plate.

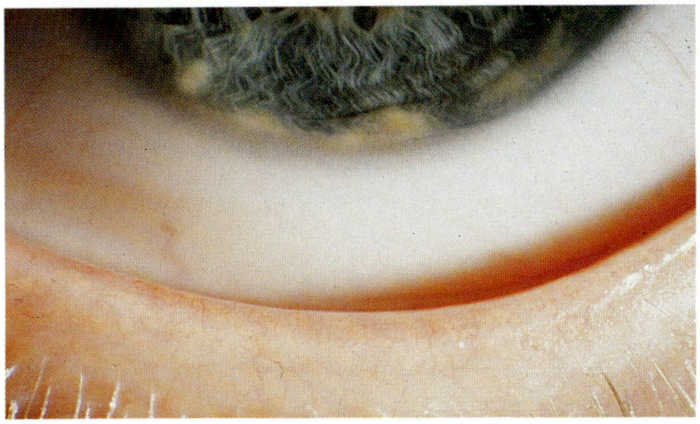

Fig. 2.1.3 The muco-cutaneous junction of the lower eyelid.

The plica semilunaris and caruncle are modified conjunctival structures at the inner canthus (Fig. 2.1.4). Here also the conjunctiva is mainly squamous and contains sebaceous glands and hair follicles.

Melanocytes are found in the basal cells of the conjunctival epithelium, as are Langerhans cells. Macrophages are numerous in the limbal region, and the sub-epithelial conjunctiva is rich in mast cells and other mediators of the immune response, forming the conjunctiva-associated lymphoid tissue (CALT).

The blood supply of the conjunctiva is derived from the palpebral and anterior ciliary arteries. They form a rich superficial plexus at the limbus. The ophthalmic division of the trigeminal nerve supplies the superior conjunctiva via its frontal and lacrimal branches. The inferior conjunctiva is innervated by the infraorbital nerve.

The accessory lacrimal glands of Krause open onto the conjunctival surface in the fornices. Glands of Mainz and Wolfring produce mucin, and also lie in the fornices.

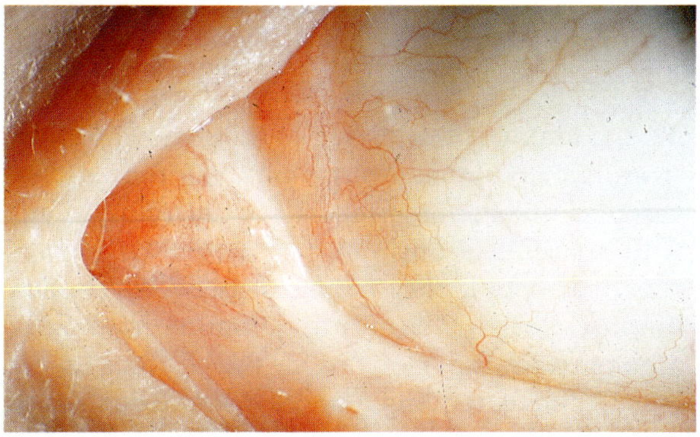

Fig. 2.1.4 The inner canthus of the right eye showing caruncle, plica, and lower punctum.

CONJUNCTIVITIS

Viral (Fig. 2.2.1)

Several viruses are capable of producing conjunctivitis either as a relatively minor feature of a systemic disease — e.g., mumps, influenza and measles — or as a characteristic ocular infection, e.g., herpes simplex, varicella-zoster, and adenovirus, often with systemic manifestations.

Viral conjunctivitis may be acute, hyperacute or chronic, and can be either unilateral or bilateral. An associated conjunctival response may be predominantly papillary, follicular, or mixed. The nature of discharge is also variable, and, though normally serous, can be purulent, membranous, or even haemorrhagic.

The symptoms of viral conjunctivitis are of mild discomfort and irritation unless accompanied by a keratitis when photophobia and reduced visual acuity may be marked. Systemic involvement can be absent, as in chronic follicular conjunctivitis associated with molluscum contagiosum infection, or severe, as in varicella-zoster or adenovirus infections.

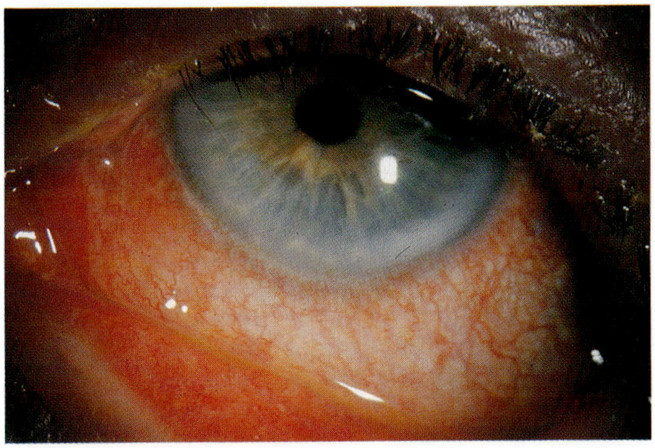

Fig. 2.2.1 Viral conjunctivitis.

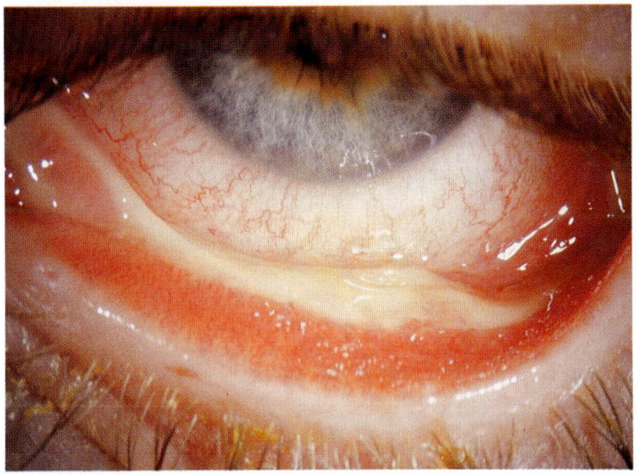

Fig. 2.2.2 Adenovirus conjunctivitis with inflammatory pseudomembrane.

Adenovirus (Fig. 2.2.2)

Adenoviruses are DNA viruses of which there are 35 immunologically distinct serotypes. Many lead to acute conjunctivitis, often with an associated pseudomembrane composed of fibrinous exudate. Certain of these viruses are notorious for producing severe epidemics of conjunctivitis, often associated with marked keratitis.

Types 3, 4 and 7 are associated with a systemic illness with fever, pharyngitis and regional lymphadenopathy, and a follicular conjunctivitis which is occasionally haemorrhagic.

Types 5, 8, 19 and, in particular, 10, cause epidemic keratoconjunctivitis where the follicular conjunctivitis is accompanied initially by a superficial epithelial keratopathy. This is sometimes followed by a focal keratitis and persistent subepithelial infiltrates. The disease begins in one eye and, although it may become bilateral, affects the fellow eye less severely.

Treatment is symptomatic, although topical antibiotics are given to reduce bacterial superinfection. The virus is highly contagious, and sufferers should be warned that they are infectious for up to two weeks following resolution of the acute phase of the disease.

Haemorrhagic viral conjunctivitis (Fig. 2.2.3)

Follicular conjunctivitis associated with subconjunctival haemorrhage has been described with enterovirus type 70, as well as some of the Coxsackie viruses that make up this group of picornaviruses. The disease is self-limiting but occurs in large epidemics. Haemorrhages are also seen in conjunctivitis associated with adenovirus and some bacteria.

Molluscum contagiosum (Fig. 2.2.4)

This large poxvirus causes a characteristic chronic unilateral follicular conjunctivitis associated with an umbilicated lid margin lesion. Occasionally a severe keratitis, with corneal filaments and vascularization may complicate this infection, which responds to the excision of the lid lesion.

Herpes simplex (Fig. 2.2.5)

When primary infection with herpes simplex virus (HSV) occurs via the ocular tissues, the typical response is a follicular conjunctivitis with blepharitis. Herpetic skin lesions are found on the lid margin and around the eye. Corneal involvement ranges from a punctate epitheliopathy to classic dendritic keratitis, depending upon the host response. Treatment is with topical antiviral agents.

Chlamydial

Chlamydial ocular infection manifests as three distinct clinical entities: trachoma, ophthalmia neonatorum and adult inclusion conjunctivitis. Trachoma is discussed under cicatricial conjunctivitis.

Ophthalmia neonatorum (Fig. 2.2.6)

During the second stage of labour, direct inoculation of the eyes of the neonate with chlamydial organisms from the cervix leads to conjunctivitis in the first week of life. There is a marked mucopurulent conjunctivitis with lid oedema and papillary hypertrophy but no follicular response. It is important to exclude gonococcal conjunctivitis by examination of conjunctival scrapings and culture. Ophthalmia neonatorum can also be caused by infection with other bacteria, herpes simplex and chemical prophylaxis.

Untreated, a trachoma-like corneal pannus may develop, and the child is at risk of chlamydial pneumonitis. Systemic therapy with erythromycin for 14 days is recommended, with or without topical tetracycline. It is important to treat the mother and her partner.

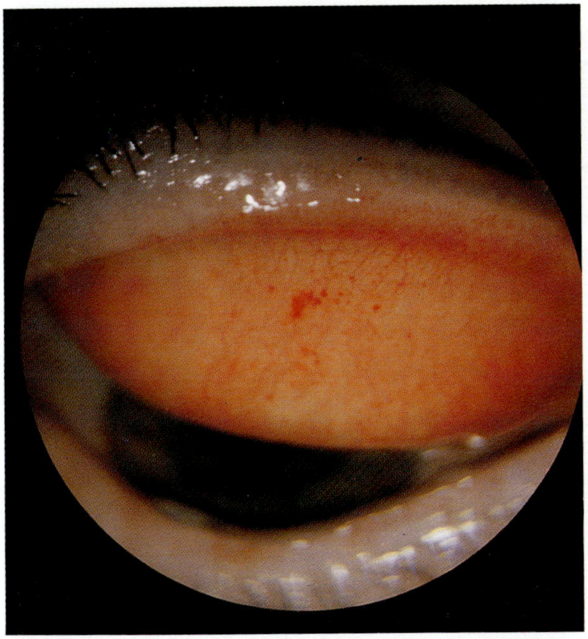

Fig. 2.2.3 Haemorrhagic viral conjunctivitis (courtesy of Mr A. B. Tullo).

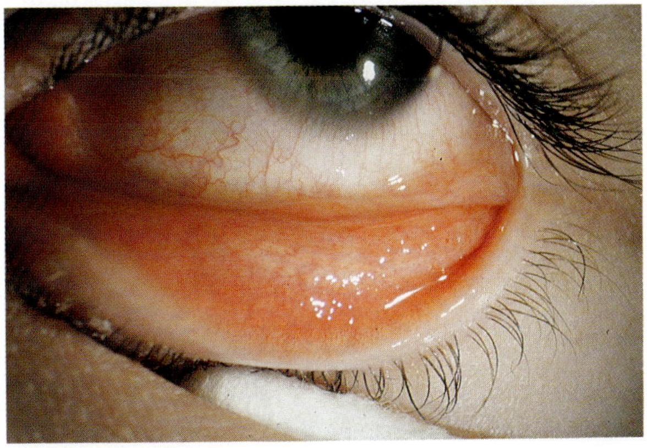

Fig. 2.2.4 Follicular conjunctivitis secondary to molluscum contagiosum infection.

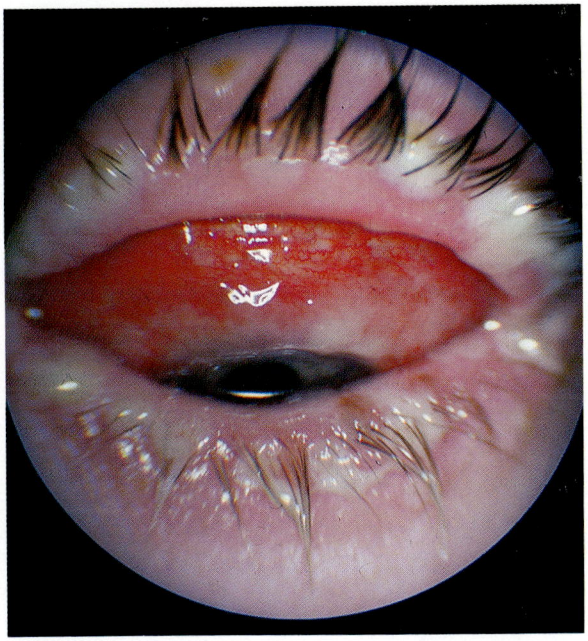

Fig. 2.2.5 Herpes simplex keratoconjunctivitis with associated blepharitis.

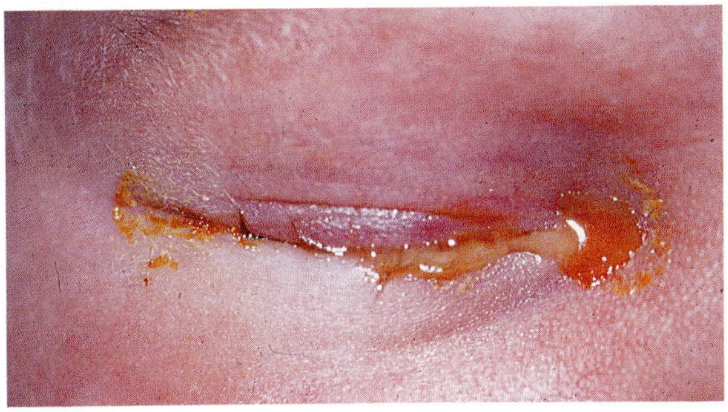

Fig. 2.2.6 Ophthalmia neonatorum due to *Chlamydia* infection.

Adult inclusion conjunctivitis (Fig. 2.2.7)

Ocular infection in the adult is a sexually transmitted disease with genital to ocular transmission by the fingers. A unilateral, subacute, follicular conjunctivitis characteristically develops 5 days after exposure. There is a purulent discharge and non-tender pre-auricular lymphadenopathy. Corneal involvement may be mild, with a fine epithelial keratopathy, or severe, with large sub-epithelial infiltrates (Fig. 2.2.8).

It is important to investigate these patients and their sexual partners for genital infection which requires treatment even if asymptomatic. The ocular infection should be treated with topical tetracycline.

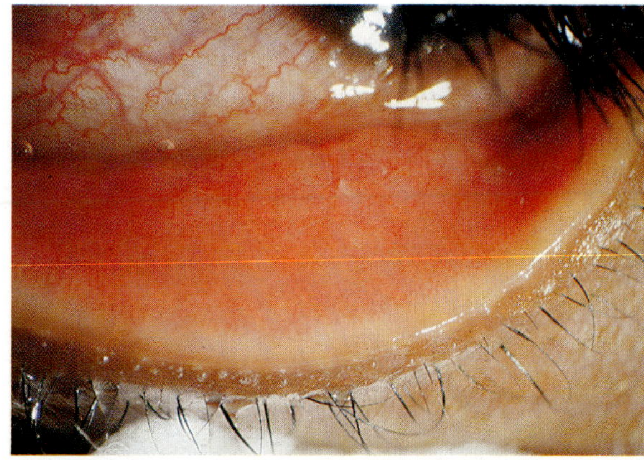

Fig. 2.2.7 Adult inclusion conjunctivitis.

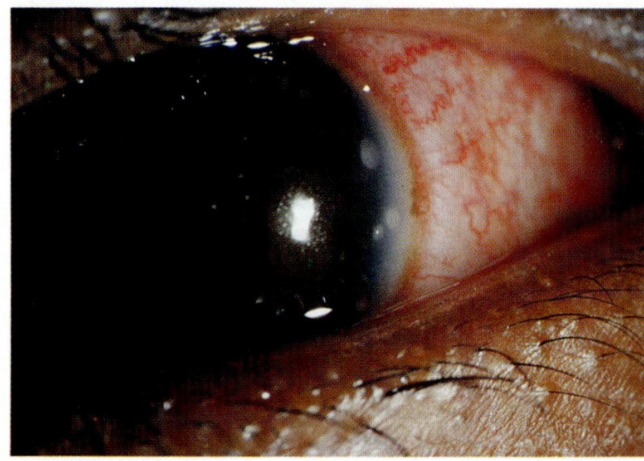

Fig. 2.2.8 Subepithelial infiltrates in *Chlamydia* infection.

Bacterial (Fig. 2.2.9)

A wide variety of bacteria are capable of producing conjunctivitis, and the disease is usually self-limiting with few ocular sequelae.

The onset is abrupt, with a purulent discharge and associated blepharitis, but no systemic involvement or lymphadenopathy. If the conjunctivitis is hyperacute with a severe response — haemorrhages, chemosis and pseudomembrane formation, but no follicles — then it is important to exclude infection with *Neisseria gonorrhoeae*.

Topical antibiotic therapy will hasten resolution of the infection, and culture and sensitivities of the responsible organism are essential only if the course becomes protracted. These should be undertaken after a period without therapy.

If conjunctivitis is recurrent, attention must be paid to the eyelids, for chronic staphylococcal blepharitis or lid malpositions, and to the tear drainage system for possible obstruction.

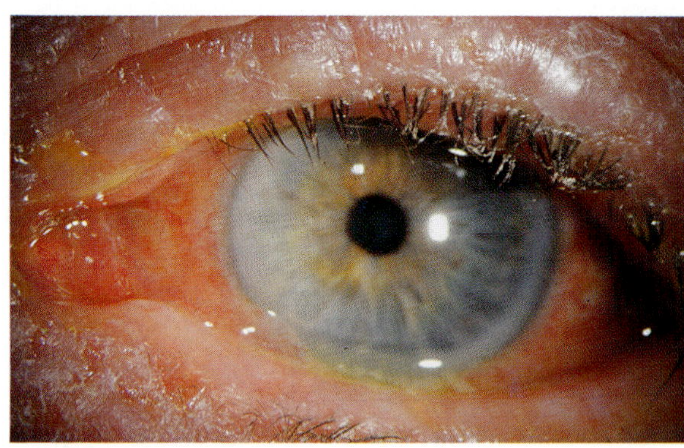

Fig. 2.2.9 Bacterial conjunctivitis with chronic staphylococcal blepharitis.

THE DRY EYE

The tear film consists of three layers: lipid, aqueous and mucin. The integrity of the tear film is dependent upon all these layers, and an abnormality or deficiency of any one will lead to the symptoms of dry eye: burning, irritation and foreign body sensation.

Lipid abnormalities

The lipid layer is derived from the meibomian glands and may be abnormal in patients with chronic meibomitis or meibomian seborrhoea. Thus, patients with blepharitis frequently have an unstable tear film and dry eye symptoms. This instability can be assessed by measuring how long it takes for breaks to appear in a fluorescein-stained tear film whilst the eyes are kept open. This is known as the tear break-up time (BUT) and should be normally longer than 10 seconds (Fig. 2.3.1).

The test is best repeated twice, ensuring that the film does not break in the same area each time, and the average time from all three tests taken.

Aqueous deficiency

Aqueous deficiency is the most common cause of a dry eye and is termed keratoconjunctivitis sicca (KCS). Usually, this is a result of involution of the main and accessory lacrimal glands, but may be associated with a variety of systemic disorders, in particular the autoimmune diseases such as rheumatoid arthritis (Fig. 2.3.2), systemic sclerosis and systemic lupus erythematosus. Autoimmune destruction of the lacrimal glands may occur in the absence of systemic disease and is termed primary Sjögrens syndrome. The term secondary Sjögrens syndrome is used to describe KCS associated with a systemic disorder.

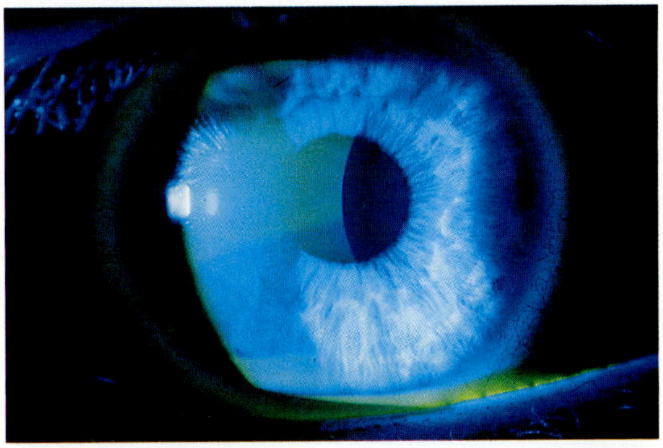

Fig. 2.3.1 Commencement of break-up of the tear film.

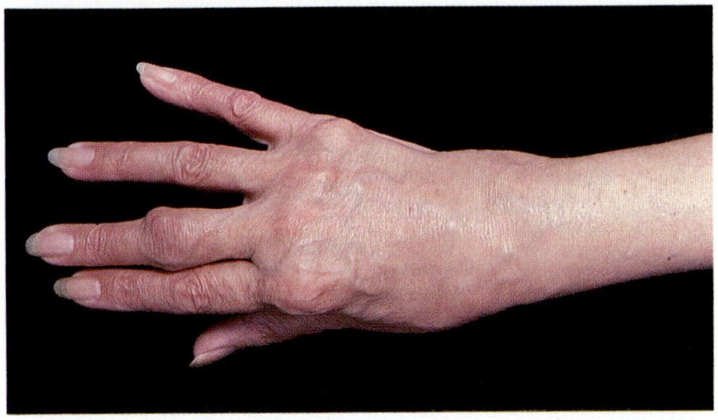

Fig. 2.3.2 Typical hand deformity in rheumatoid arthritis (courtesy of Dr Amos).

Mucin deficiency

Destruction of the mucin-producing conjunctival goblet cells leads to a dry eye because of poor wetting of the corneal and conjunctival surfaces. Mucin deficiency can be caused by cicatricial conjunctivitis and by vitamin A deficiency.

Hypovitaminosis A is usually part of a generally poor nutritional state but may be an isolated deficiency in people taking an unusual diet. Vitamin A is essential for normal differentiation of epithelial surfaces and a deficiency leads to keratinization of the cornea and the conjunctiva. Bitot's spot is a chalky keratinization of the conjunctiva (Fig. 2.3.3), classically associated with vitamin A deficiency, but which can be seen in other conditions causing severe drying of the eye (xerophthalmia) (Fig. 2.3.4). Progression can lead to corneal melting, which is termed keratomalacia, and subsequent perforation.

Investigations

The symptoms of burning and foreign body sensation are usually enough to suggest dry eye, but several investigations are useful in confirming the diagnosis and assessing the severity of the condition.

Examination

The tear film is contaminated, and in aqueous deficiency states mucin may be present in large amounts leading to filamentary keratitis (Fig. 2.3.5). The tear meniscus between the lid margin and cornea is reduced or absent. Rose Bengal introduced into the tear film will readily stain cornea and conjunctiva, particularly in the interpalpebral area (Fig. 2.3.6). The tear break-up time (BUT) has been discussed earlier.

Schirmer's test (Fig. 2.3.7)

Several Schirmer's tests are described. All involve the placement of a filter paper strip into the inferior fornix and measurement of the length of paper wetted over a five-minute period. Wetting of less than 5 mm is considered abnormal.

Enzyme assay

The lacrimal gland produces several enzymes and proteins which are absent or reduced in KCS. Both tear lysozyme and lactoferrin can be measured to give a quantitative assessment of tear deficiency.

Tear osmolarity

Tears are collected in a micropipette and osmolarity measured by a freezing point method. Dry eyes have a tear osmolarity of greater than 312 mmol.

Impression cytology

Superficial conjunctival cells can be biopsied by applying a micropore filter paper to the surface of the anaesthetized eye, and staining the attached cells with a modified Papanicolau stain. This technique can be used to assess goblet cell density, which is reduced in dry eyes, and conjunctival keratinization, which is increased in dry eyes.

Treatment

When a systemic disease is associated with dry eye, it is important to diagnose accurately and treat this disease. Treatment of the systemic condition, however, rarely has a significant influence upon the dry eye.

Blepharitis, if present, must be treated, and any local cause of tear film irregularity such as trichiasis or entropion should be corrected.

The mainstay of treatment is the frequent use of topical lubricants, of which there are many. Patients will often prefer the use of one over another similar preparation, for no apparent reason, and therefore several should be tried. The preservatives used in these preparations are toxic to epithelia, and some patients are particularly sensitive. Preservative-free preparations are indicated in such cases.

Slow-release lubricants such as lacriserts can be of value in those who are unable to use dropper bottles because of arthritis (Fig. 2.3.8). Rarely, an extremely dry eye needs to be irrigated using an appropriately designed pump mechanism fitted to a pair of glasses.

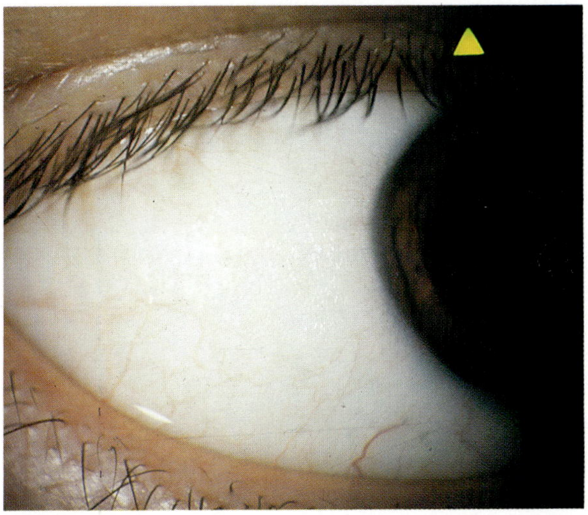

Fig. 2.3.3 Bitot's spot.

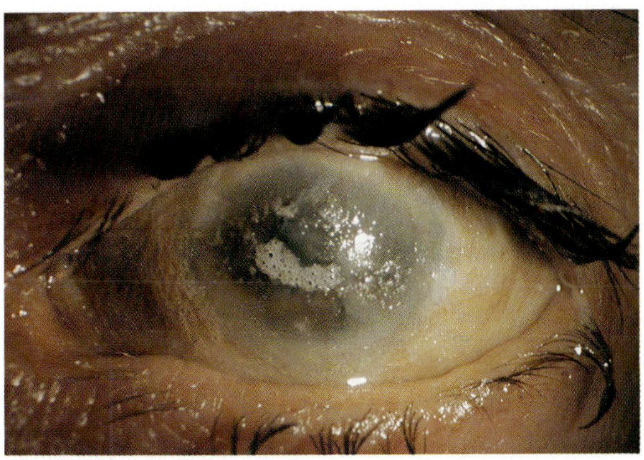

Fig. 2.3.4 Xerophthalmia.

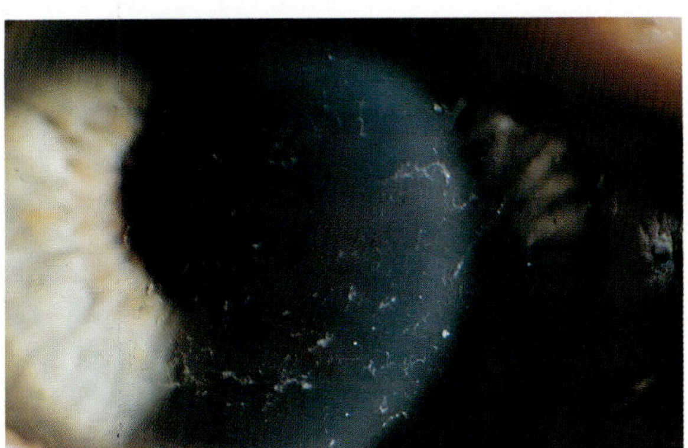

Fig. 2.3.5 Filamentary keratitis.

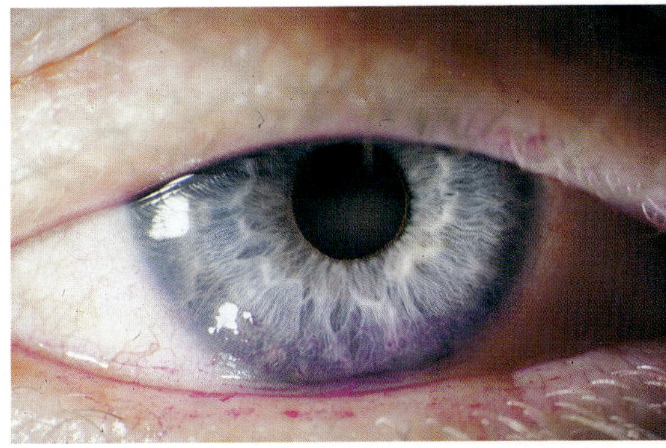

Fig. 2.3.6 Rose Bengal staining of the cornea and conjunctiva in keratoconjunctivitis sicca.

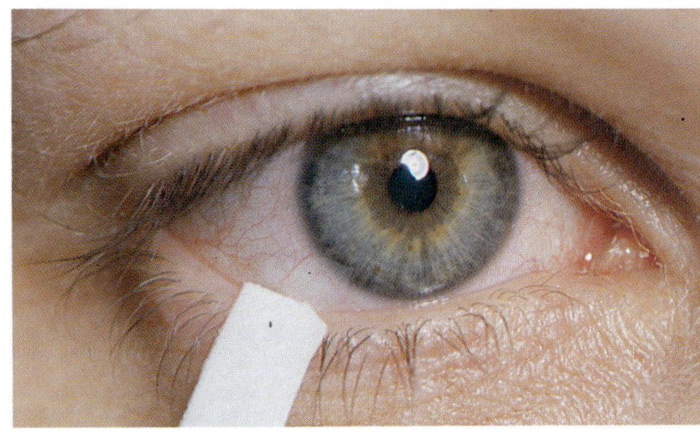

Fig. 2.3.7 Schirmer's test.

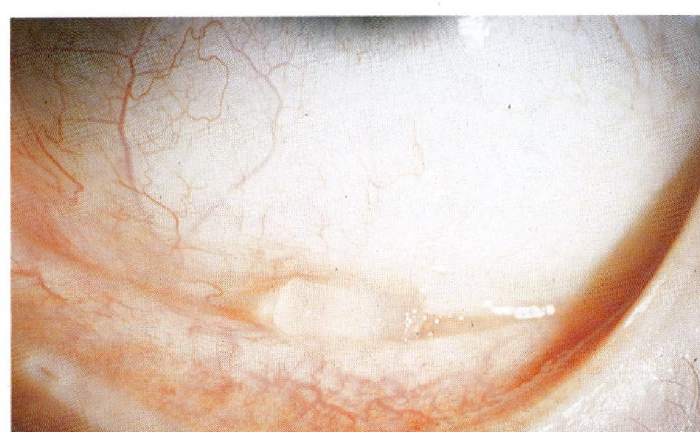

Fig. 2.3.8 Lacrisert positioned in the lower fornix.

Tear conservation can be attempted by occluding the lacrimal puncta and canaliculi. This can be achieved either temporarily with gelatin or collagen rods inserted into the canaliculi (Fig. 2.3.9) or punctal plugs (Fig. 2.3.10a and b) or permanently with canalicular cautery (Fig. 2.3.11). It is important to occlude the puncta temporarily prior to any irreversible procedure, in order to ensure that epiphora does not develop. Evaporation of the tear film may be reduced by wearing goggles or humidifying the environment.

Topical mucolytics, such as acetylcysteine, can be of value when excess mucus is present. Filamentary keratitis may be resistant to therapy and a therapeutic soft contact lens may be required. The use of contact lenses in dry eye states is prone to infection, however, and close supervision is required.

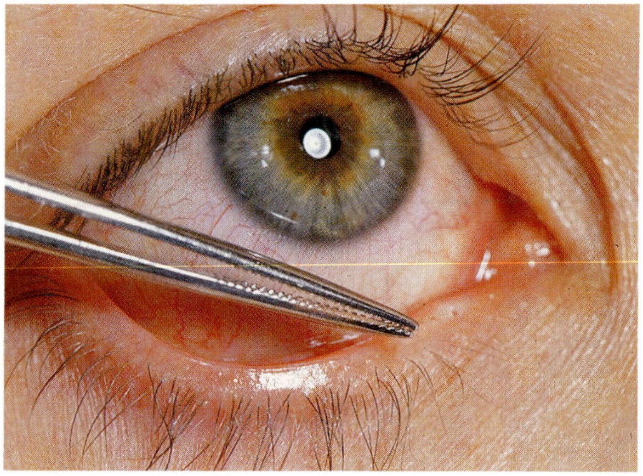

Fig. 2.3.9 Temporary punctal occlusion with gelatin rods.

a

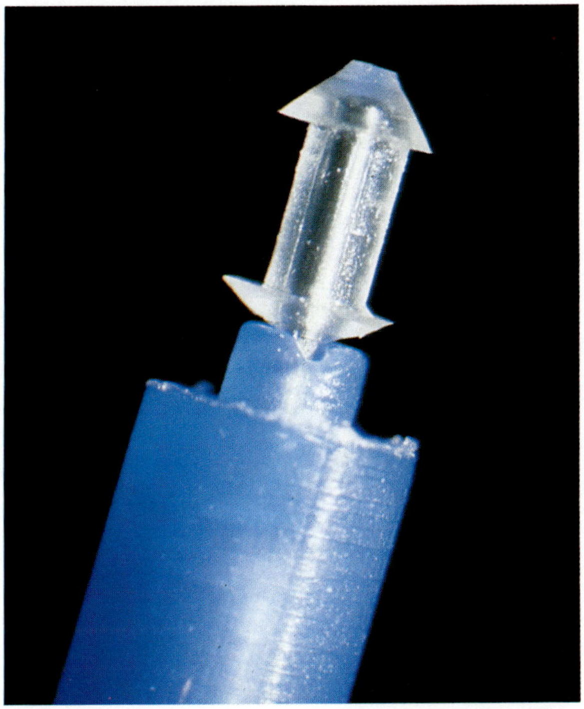

b

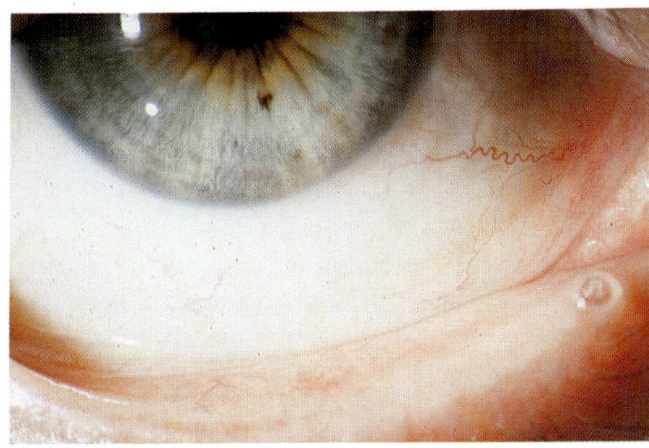

Fig. 2.3.10 Punctal plug (**b**), and punctal plug in position (**b**).

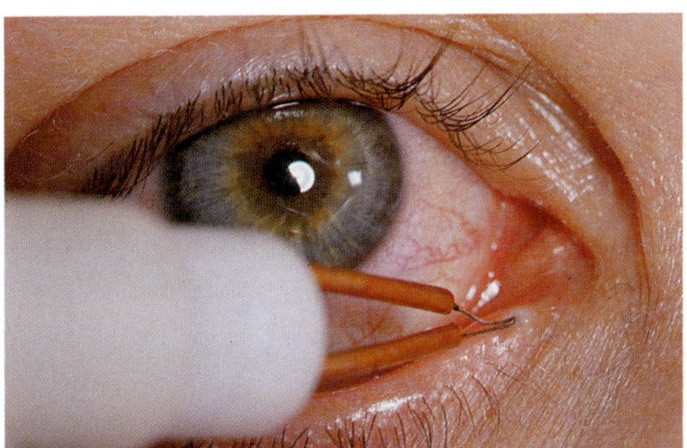

Fig. 2.3.11 Canalicular cautery.

CICATRICIAL CONJUNCTIVITIS

Chronic, recurrent conjunctivitis associated with sub-epithelial scarring can lead to dry eyes, entropion and trichiasis, corneal and conjunctival keratinization, corneal vascularization, scarring and perforation. This collection of features comprises cicatricial conjunctivitis (Fig. 2.4.1), which has a number of aetiologies. Mild degrees are seen in patients with blepharitis and following viral conjunctivitis, whereas more severe disease occurs in trachoma, the bullous dermatoses, atopic disease, drug therapy and following chemical burns.

Trachoma

This chlamydial infection is endemic in Africa, the Middle East, India and Southeast Asia. An active infectious stage occurs in children as a follicular and papillary conjunctivitis, often complicated by secondary bacterial infection. After 10–20 years, the scarring associated with repeated infections leads to corneal opacification.

The MacCallan classification of trachoma recognizes four stages of the disease. Stage I is characterized by a follicular and mild papillary conjunctivitis with only a mild superficial keratitis. In Stage II(a) tarsal and limbal follicles are predominant; these are replaced by papillae in Stage II(b). Corneal pannus and sub-epithelial infiltrates are found in Stage II (Fig. 2.4.2). The limbal follicles of Stage II disease necrose to leave Herbert's pits.

Conjunctival scarring is the predominant feature of Stage III disease, typically seen as a horizontal band in the tarsal conjunctiva called Arlt's line (Fig. 2.4.3).

Stage IV disease comprises a dry eye state with corneal vascularization, and scarring, entropion and trichiasis.

Treatment of trachoma is with systemic tetracycline, erythromycin or sulphonamide in the acute phase. Late disease management should be directed towards the surgical correction of entropion and trichiasis, together with tear film replacements.

Bullous dermatoses

These are a group of autoimmune disorders involving the skin and mucous membranes, including the conjunctiva. Each dermatosis has characteristic immunopathological features, but there is considerable overlap between the clinical signs.

Pemphigus (Fig. 2.4.4)

In pemphigus there are circulating antibodies to the intercellular determinants of the epidermis. The skin lesion is of thin-walled blisters which easily rupture, although scarring is not a major feature (Fig. 2.4.5). Ocular involvement, which comprises corneal and conjunctival blisters and erosions, is uncommon.

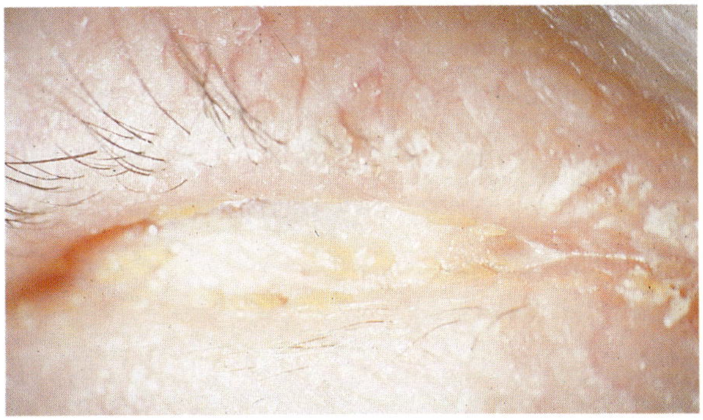

Fig. 2.4.1 End-stage cicatricial conjunctivitis.

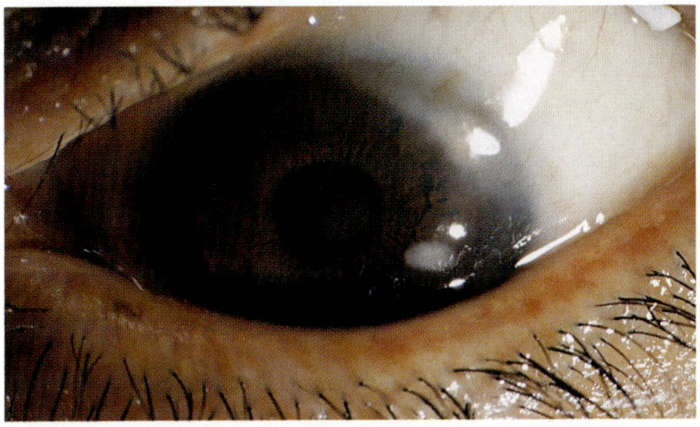

Fig. 2.4.2 Corneal pannus and sub-epithelial infiltrates in Stage II trachoma.

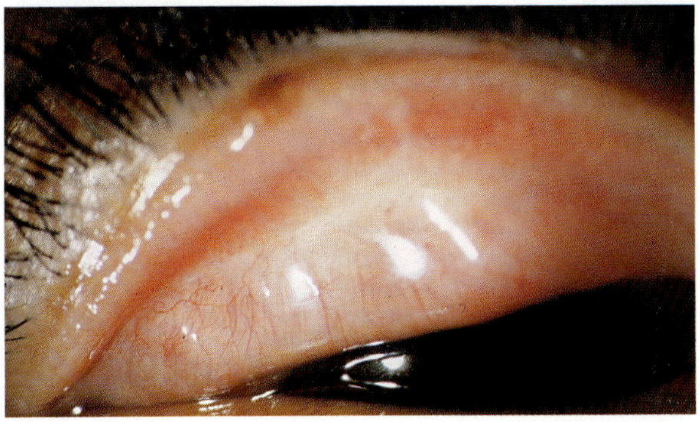

Fig. 2.4.3 Arlt's line.

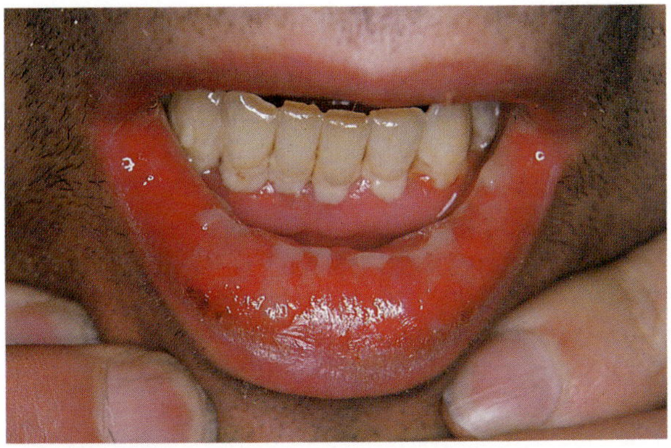

Fig. 2.4.4 Oral lesions in pemphigus (courtesy of Dr A. Messenger).

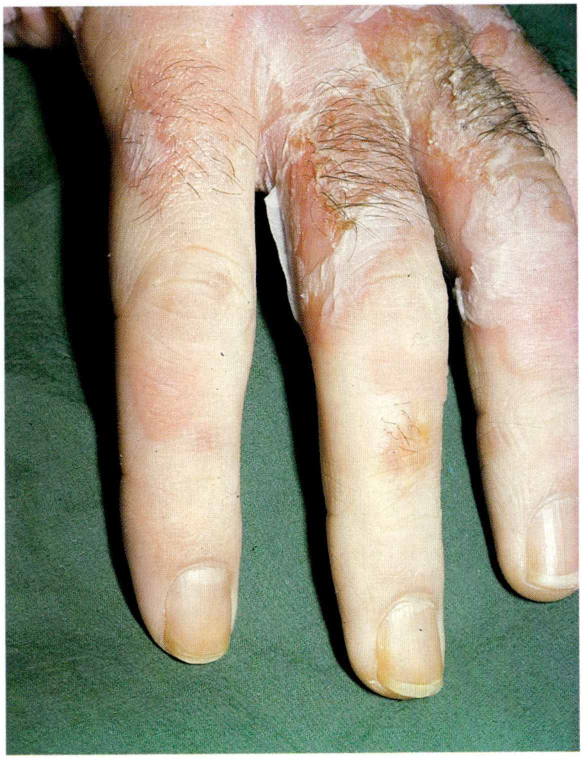

Fig. 2.4.5 Typical skin blistering in pemphigus.

Pemphigoid (Fig. 2.4.6)

Bullous pemphigoid and mucous membrane (or cicatricial) pemphigoid are similar immunologically, with antibodies found bound to the basement membrane of the epidermis or mucous membrane epithelium.

Bullous pemphigoid is characterized by thick-walled haemorrhagic blisters involving the skin with infrequent mucous membrane involvement.

In mucous membrane pemphigoid, blisters are less frequent, but scarring involves the conjunctival, oral, oesophageal and occasionally anal and genital mucous membranes.

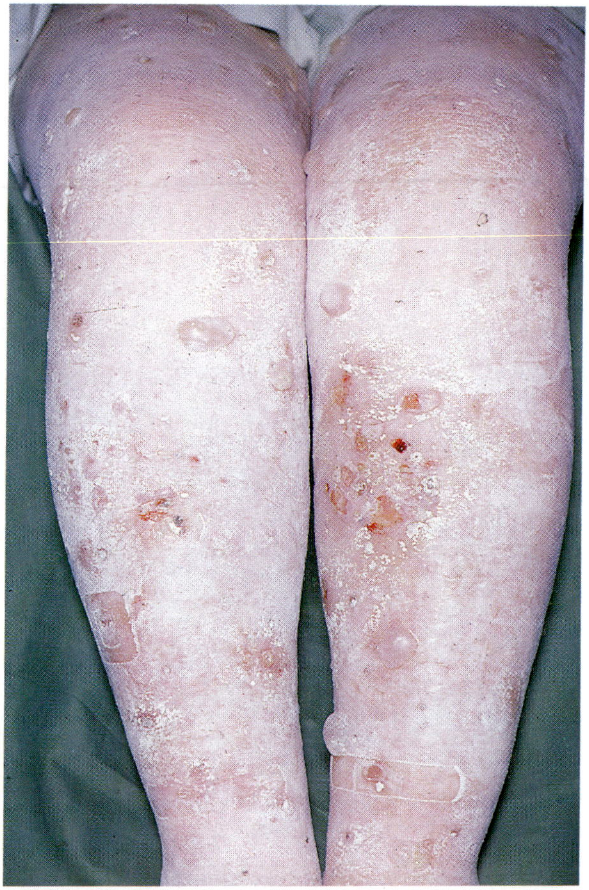

Fig. 2.4.6 Skin blisters in bullous pemphigoid (courtesy of Dr A. Messenger).

Dermatitis herpetiformis (Fig. 2.4.7)

This condition demonstrates a papillary deposit of IgA in the basement membrane. Clinically, the lesions are typically vesicular, but can appear identical to bullous pemphigoid or mucous membrane pemphigoid. Sometimes the IgA is deposited in a continuous manner in the basement membrane, a disorder termed 'linear IgA disease'.

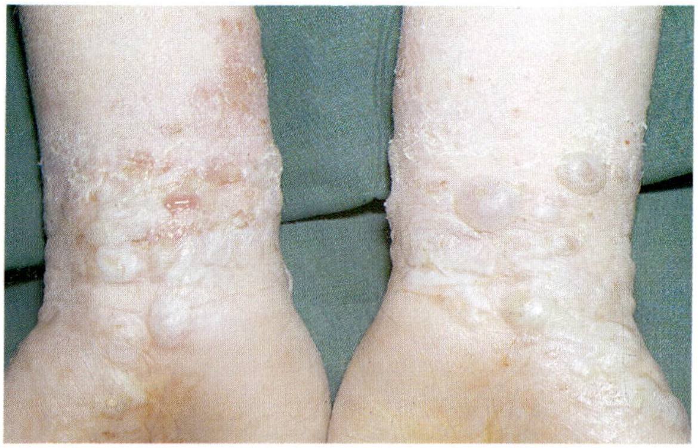

Fig. 2.4.7 Bullous eruption on wrists in dermatitis herpetiformis (courtesy of Dr A. Messenger).

Stevens–Johnson syndrome

This is a systemic disease which usually follows drug therapy or an infective illness. A skin eruption occurs which is vesico-bullous, typically a target or iris lesion (erythema multiforme) (Fig. 2.4.8). Mucous membrane involvement is common, especially in the mouth (Fig. 2.4.9). Immune complexes can be demonstrated in blood vessels in the dermis.

Ocular features

The conjunctival features of all the bullous dermatoses are similar. There is a mucous conjunctivitis during the acute phase of the condition (Fig. 2.4.10), with sometimes blisters and ulcers found on the conjunctival surface.

Fine subepithelial fibrosis develops on the tarsal conjunctival surface (Fig. 2.4.11), and there is loss of definition of the plica and caruncle (Fig. 2.4.12).

The fornices lose volume, and adhesions termed 'symblephara' form between the bulbar and palpebral conjunctiva (Fig. 2.4.13).

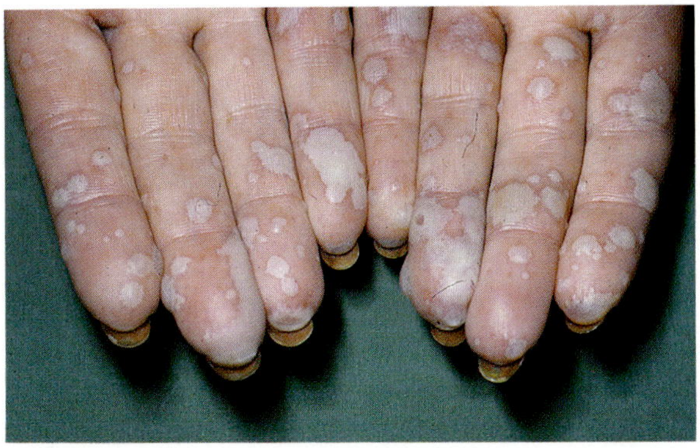

Fig. 2.4.8 Vesico-bullous skin eruption in Stevens–Johnson syndrome (courtesy of Dr A. Messenger).

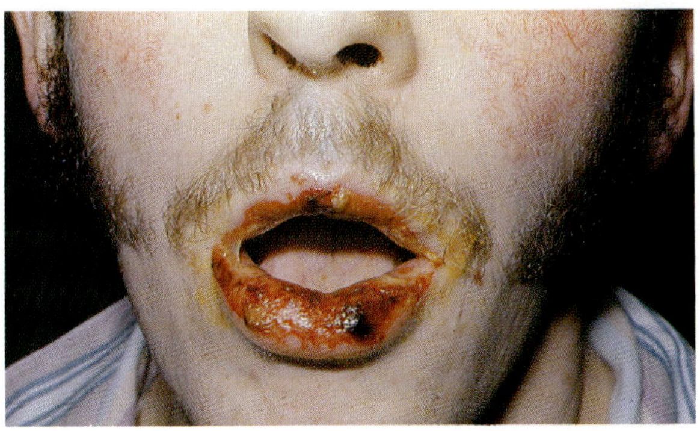

Fig. 2.4.9 Oral mucosal involvement in Stevens–Johnson syndrome.

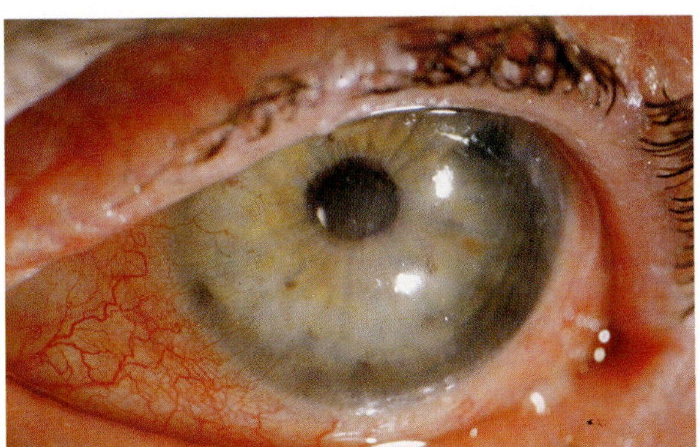

Fig. 2.4.10 Mucous conjunctivitis in acute mucous membrane pemphigoid.

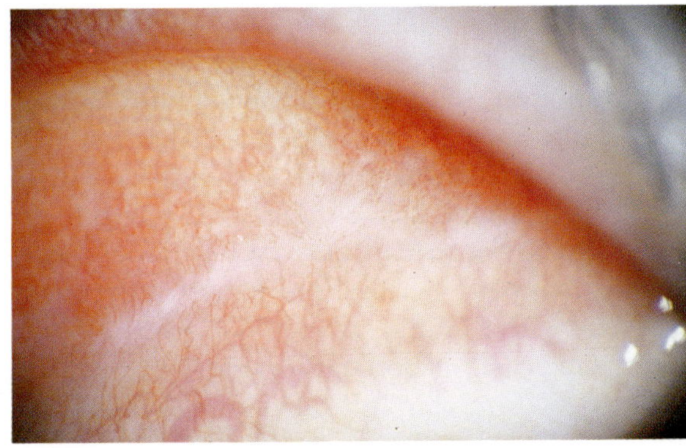

Fig. 2.4.11 Subepithelial fibrosis in mucous membrane pemphigoid.

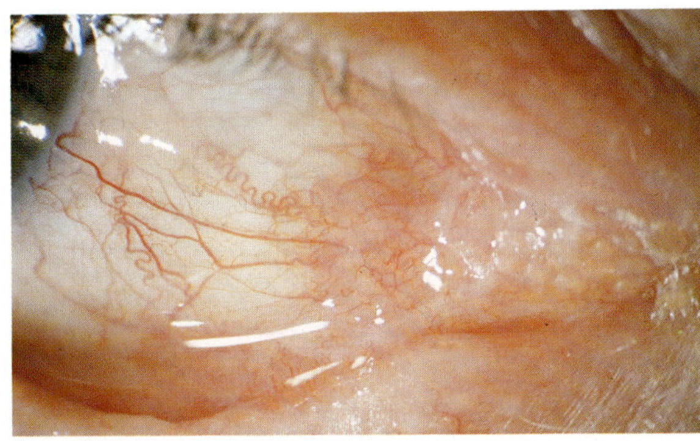

Fig. 2.4.12 Loss of medial canthal architecture in mucous membrane pemphigoid.

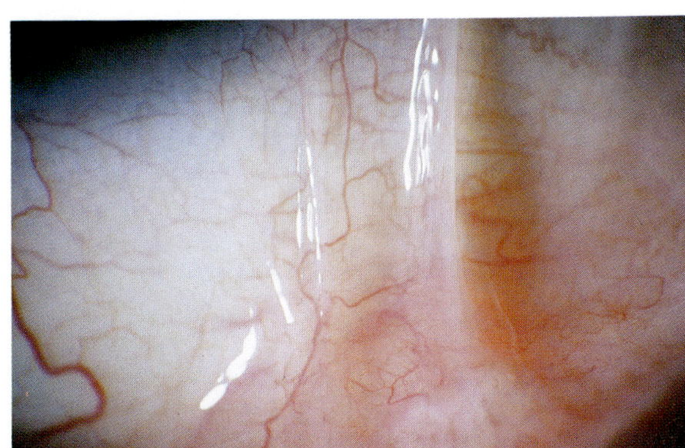

Fig. 2.4.13 Symblepharon.

Loss of goblet cells and scarring of the orifices of the lacrimal glands contribute to a dry eye. Keratinization of the conjunctival and corneal epithelium then follows (Fig. 2.4.14).

Cicatricial entropion and trichiasis combined with the extreme xerosis lead to corneal vascularization, scarring and ulceration. Spontaneous corneal perforation is not infrequent. The end stage of the disease is a non-inflamed keratinized opaque corneal surface with complete absence of fornices. Adhesion of lid margins is termed ankyloblepharon.

Treatment

It is essential to recognize these chronic progressive conjunctival inflammations early in order for treatment to modify the potentially poor prognosis.

Acute episodes should be treated with systemic immunosuppressive agents such as cyclophosphamide or azathioprine, either alone or in combination with systemic steroid. Dapsone and cyclosporin are also effective.

Supportive local treatment should include lubricants, treatment of secondary infection and surgical correction of lid abnormalities.

Keratinization responds to topical retinoid therapy (Fig. 2.4.15a and b). Topical steroids are of benefit in the acute phase of Stevens–Johnson syndrome, which, unlike the other bullous dermatoses, does not progress once the initial episode has resolved.

Drug-induced cicatricial conjunctivitis (Fig. 2.4.16)

In addition to the condition of drug-induced Stevens–Johnson syndrome, several systemic and topical drugs can produce conjunctival scarring.

Oral practolol use led to a number of patients developing mucous membrane scarring followed by dry eyes. Some topical preparations used in glaucoma management can produce changes similar to those seen in the bullous dermatoses.

Chemical burns (Fig. 2.4.17)

Chemical burns, and in particular those from alkalis, can cause progressive conjunctival scarring, with symblepharon formation, dry eye, and chronic corneal epithelial disease.

Acute burns require topical steroid therapy and antibiotics together with vitamin C supplements. Collagenase inhibitors such as cystine are useful in the treatment of corneal melting. Chronic epithelial disease may require treatment with a bandage contact lens, conjunctival flap or epithelial graft.

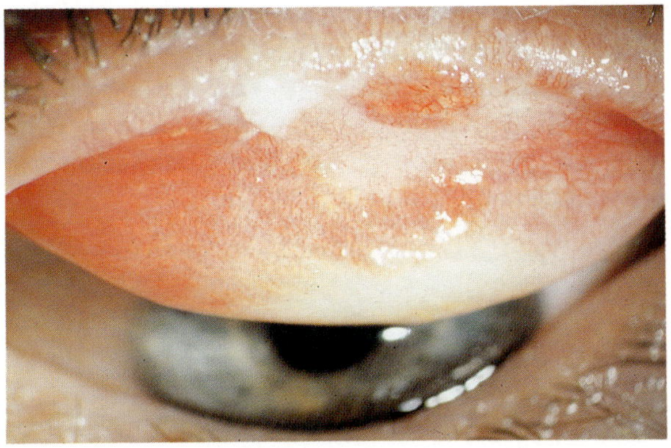

Fig. 2.4.14 Conjunctival keratinization secondary to Stevens–Johnson syndrome.

a

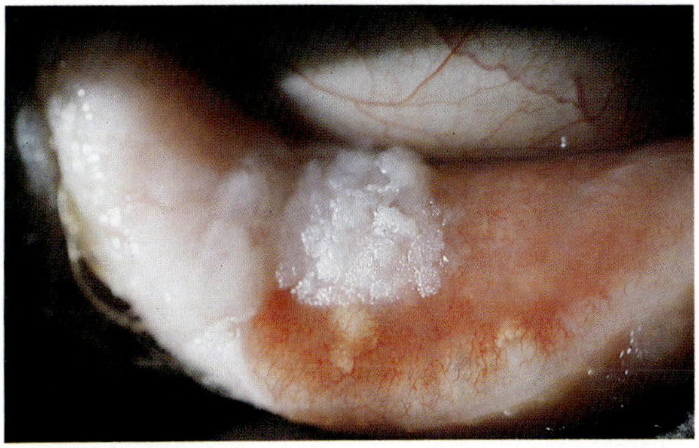

b

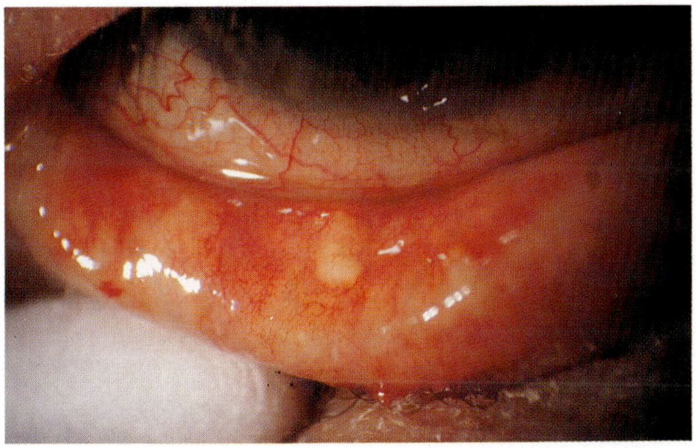

Fig. 2.4.15 Keratinization of the conjuctiva before (**a**) and after (**b**) topical retinoic acid.

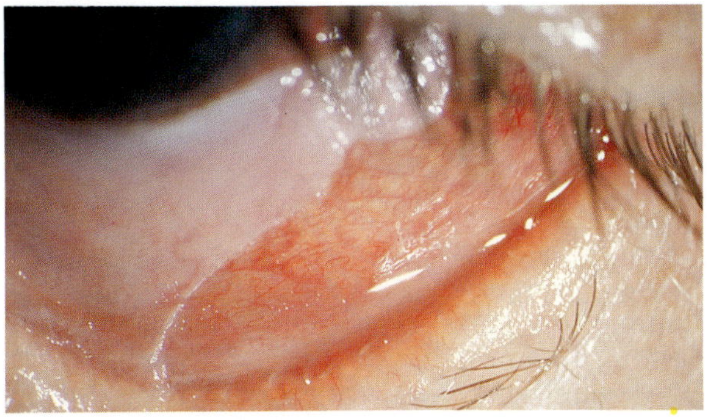

Fig. 2.4.16 Drug-induced conjunctival cicatrization with marked squamous metaplasia.

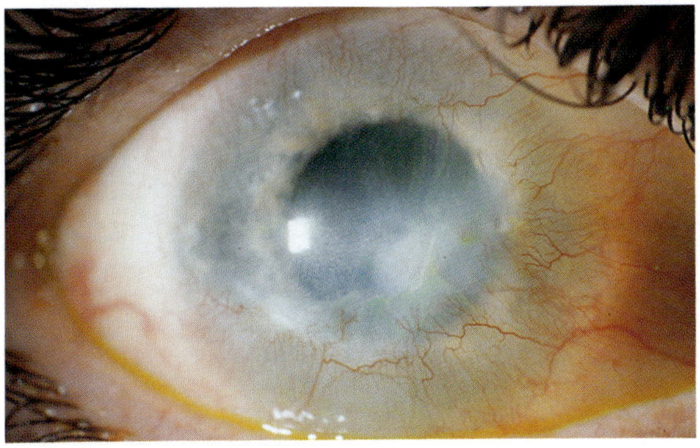

Fig. 2.4.17 Chemical burn.

BENIGN CONJUNCTIVAL LESIONS

Haemangioma (Fig. 2.5.1)

This rare hamartomatous lesion is benign, and usually regresses spontaneously. It is usually present at birth, or shortly after, and may grow quite actively in early childhood. Excision is required only occasionally for cosmetic reasons.

Conjunctival cyst (Fig. 2.5.2)

A cyst of the conjunctiva full of clear fluid commonly follows minor local trauma or surgery. It requires removal only if symptomatic. Simple puncturing of the cyst often leads to recurrence, and complete excision is preferable.

Papilloma

Conjunctival papillomata occur most frequently at the inner canthus (Fig. 2.5.3), but may be more extensive (Fig. 2.5.4). They usually occur in children and young adults following papova virus infection. Simple excision is adequate for the majority of lesions, although cryotherapy may be required for more extensive or recurrent disease. Surgical debulking together with application of dinitrochlorobenzene has also been used.

Pinguecula (Fig. 2.5.5)

This common lesion presents in the interpalpebral zone of the conjunctiva as a yellowish elevation, and consists of degenerate subepithelial collagen, often associated with calcification. No treatment is required, although some pingueculae progress to pterygia formation.

Pterygium (Fig. 2.5.6)

This is a fibrovascular proliferation of conjunctiva, situated in the interpalpebral zone, most commonly on the nasal side, which grows across the limbus to invade the corneal stroma. The condition is common in hot, dry climates, being predisposed to by ultraviolet radiation and drying of the tear film. Treatment is the symptomatic relief of any consequent tear film disturbance using topical lubricants. Surgical excision is required if the growth extends towards the visual axis. Adjunctive cautery, β-irradiation and administration of thiotepa or topical corticosteroid have all been used to try and lessen the high recurrence rate.

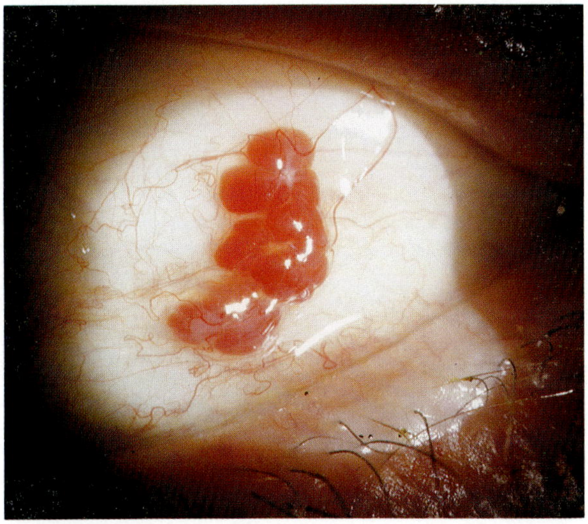

Fig. 2.5.1 Conjunctival haemangioma.

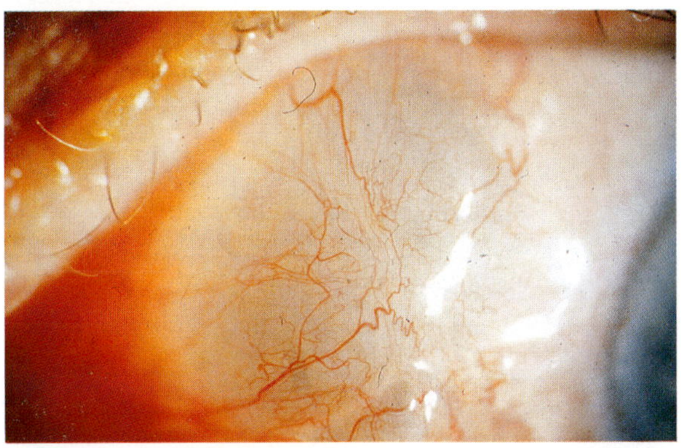

Fig. 2.5.2 Conjunctival cyst.

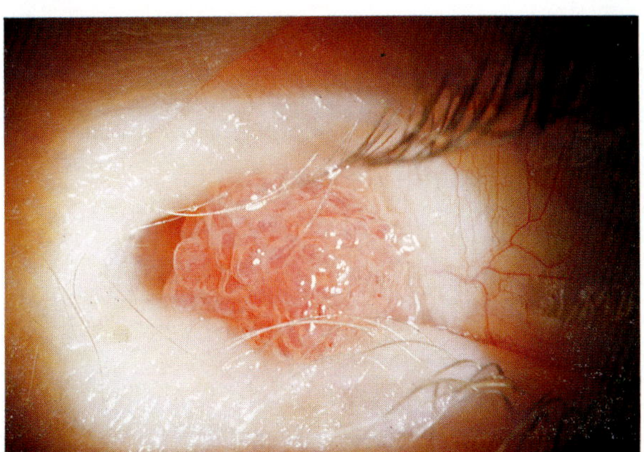

Fig. 2.5.3 Conjunctival papilloma situated at inner canthus.

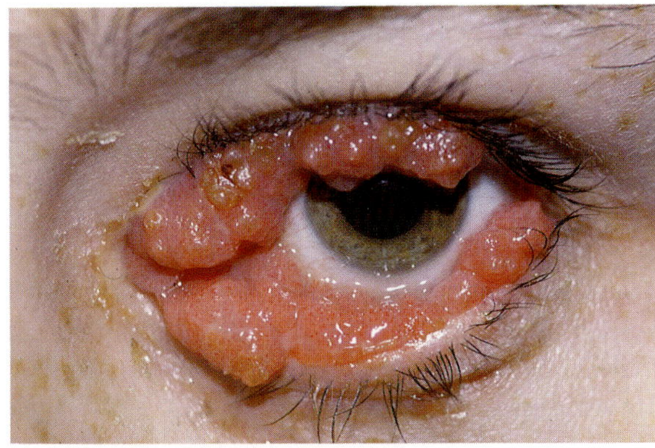

Fig. 2.5.4 Gross conjunctival papillomatosis.

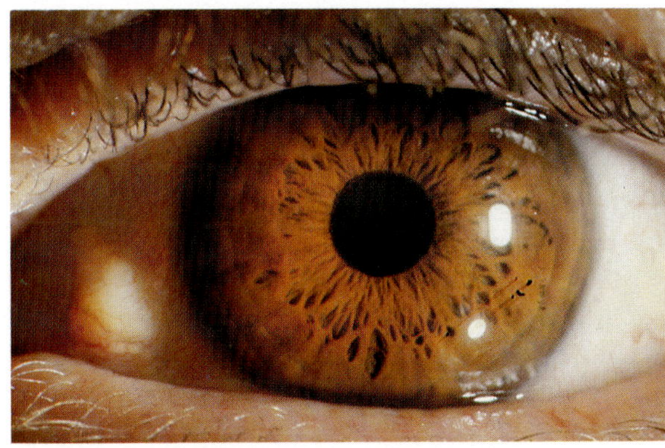

Fig. 2.5.5 Pinguecula situated in the nasal interpalpebral conjunctiva.

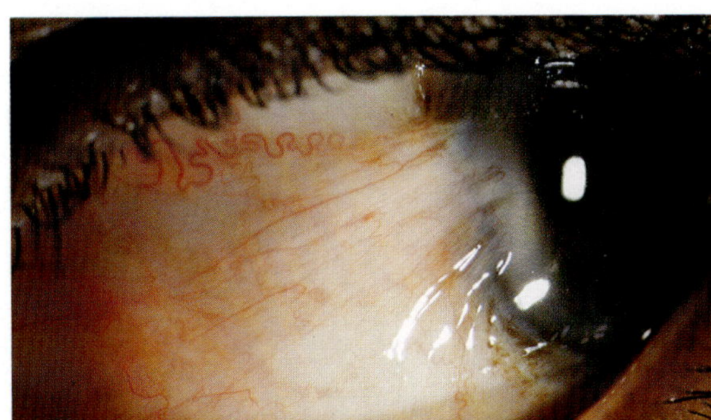

Fig. 2.5.6 Early pterygium.

Phlycten (Fig. 2.5.7)

This is a manifestation of delayed hypersensitivity to bacterial antigen, following infection classically with tuberculosis, but more commonly with staphylococci. It presents as a small, elevated white nodule near, or at, the limbus, with surrounding conjunctival inflammation. It is most common in children. The nodule develops into a microabscess which then heals, usually about two weeks after onset. A short course of topical steroid hastens the resolution, and should be combined with treatment of any concurrent blepharitis, which predisposes to the condition.

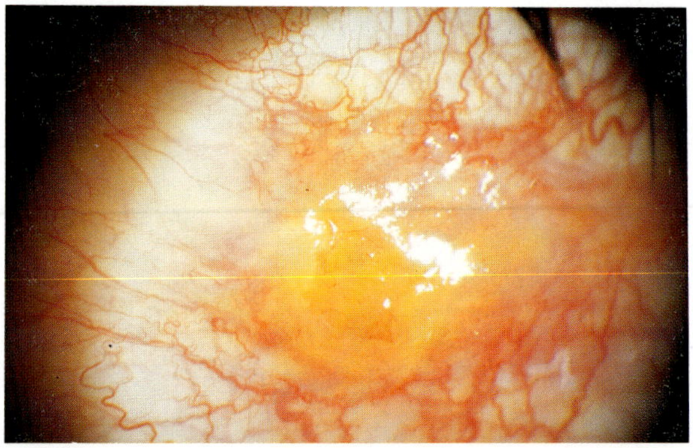

Fig. 2.5.7 Phlycten with surrounding conjunctival inflammation.

Sarcoid granuloma (Fig. 2.5.8)

This may be the only ocular manifestation of systemic sarcoidosis, and biopsy is often a useful confirmation of the diagnosis. 'Blind' conjunctival biopsy in suspected sarcoidosis, in the absence of any visible granulomata, yields positive results in approximately one third of patients with systemic disease, obviating the need for biopsy of less accessible tissues. In the presence of conjunctival follicles, biopsy is twice as likely to be positive.

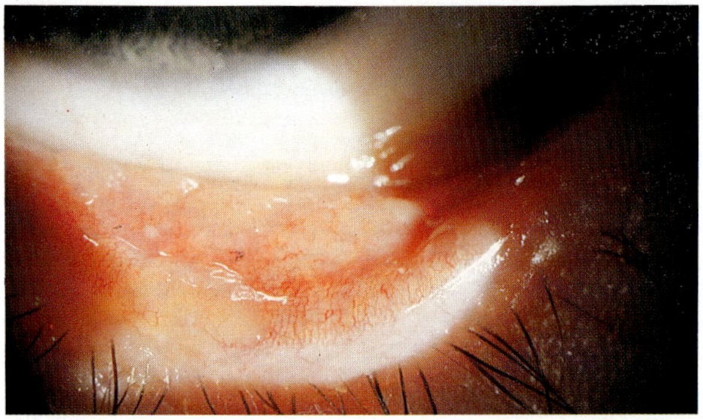

Fig. 2.5.8 Sarcoid granuloma in the palpebral conjunctiva of the lower lid.

Stitch granuloma (Fig. 2.5.9)

These occur less commonly since the refinement of suture materials, but may be both cosmetically unsightly and the cause of discomfort. Surgical excision is indicated once granulomata have become established, although topical corticosteroids may abort their evolution.

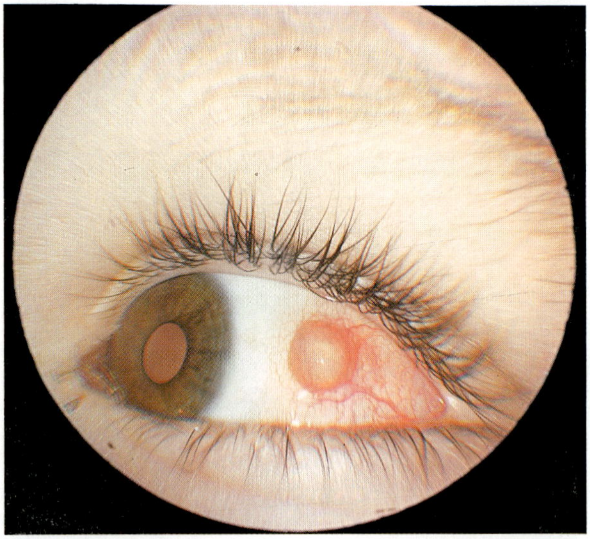

Fig. 2.5.9 Stitch granuloma following squint surgery.

PREMALIGNANT AND MALIGNANT LESIONS

Conjunctival melanosis

In children, this refers simply to an area of increased pigmentation of the conjunctiva, present since birth or an early age, and not increasing in size. It reflects excess melanin deposition, as in a skin freckle. These lesions are benign, and do not require excision (Fig. 2.6.1). The term conjunctival ephilis (freckle) is used to describe such pigmentation.

Melanosis acquired as an adult, however, in a previously normal area of conjunctiva, is termed 'conjunctival melanocytic intraepithelial neoplasia' (CMIN) (Fig. 2.6.2). The old terminology for this was 'precancerous melanosis', and reflects the progression of a proportion of these lesions to malignant melanoma. Such lesions should therefore be excised and examined histologically.

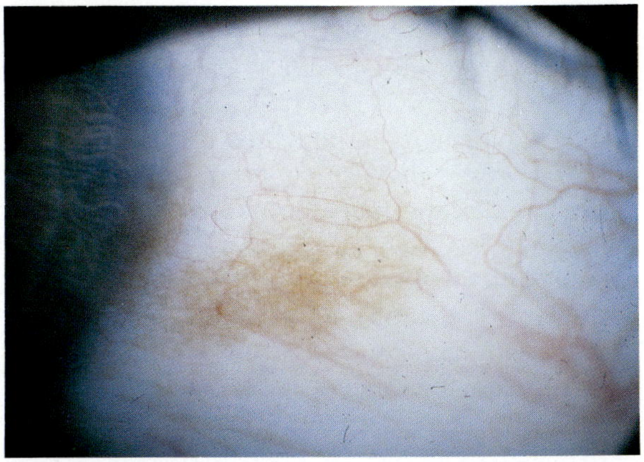

Fig. 2.6.1 Conjunctival ephilis (courtesy of Mr I. G. Rennie).

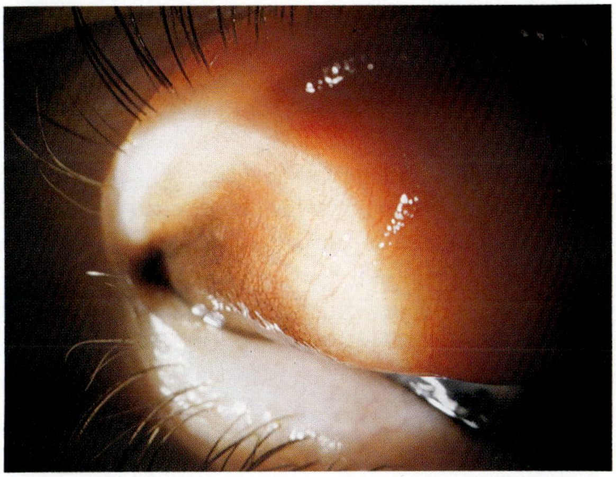

Fig. 2.6.2 Everted upper lid demonstrating acquired melanosis (CMIN) of the palpebral conjunctiva (courtesy of Mr I. G. Rennie).

Naevus

This develops from a proliferation of melanocytic cells, and occurs congenitally or in early life. Naevi are benign, although if biopsied before puberty, may show cellular mitoses at the dermis–epidermis junctional zone, suggestive of malignancy.

Such junctional activity seen in a biopsy of a naevus from an adult, however, does imply onset of malignant change. Any newly acquired naevus in adulthood, or change in size or colour of a pre-existing naevus, should therefore be biopsied. A naevus may be deeply pigmented (Fig. 2.6.3), but it more commonly appears as a lightly pigmented, cystic lesion (Fig. 2.6.4).

Squamous metaplasia (Fig. 2.6.5)

This can develop following any chronic irritative process, such as trichiasis or ultraviolet radiation, but may also arise de novo. Histologically, there is a change in the conjunctival epithelial cells from the normal columnar and cubical type, to squamous, although they remain well differentiated (Fig. 2.6.6). Squamous metaplasia may progress to carcinoma in situ, or frank squamous cell carcinoma, and therefore its identification requires careful observation.

Carcinoma in situ (Fig. 2.6.7)

This is a histological description which represents cellular atypia and abnormal mitotic activity extending throughout the thickness of the epithelium, without invasion of the substantia propria. The more recent term 'conjunctival intraepithelial neoplasia' (CIN), is used to describe both such change extending through the whole thickness of the epithelium, and that limited to partial thickness involvement. Clinically it cannot be distinguished from squamous metaplasia.

Although most CIN does not progress to squamous cell carcinoma, up to 20% of cases do become invasive. Treatment of CIN should therefore involve complete excision of the involved conjunctiva, using frozen section control, and double freeze–thaw adjunctive cryotherapy.

Squamous cell carcinoma (Fig. 2.6.8)

This invades the tissues deep to the epithelium, and may spread locally into the lids and orbit, as well as producing distant metastases.

It is predisposed to by exposure to sunlight, and may present a variety of appearances, usually beginning at the limbus. These include a papillary-type appearance, an indolent spreading form, and a gelatinous consistency. Squamous cell carcinoma may also masquerade as a unilateral chronic conjunctivitis, refractory to treatment, and such disease should therefore be biopsied or examined by exfoliative cytology.

Treatment of squamous cell carcinoma is similar to that of carcinoma in situ, unless the lesion is particularly extensive, or invades the globe, in which case either limited exenteration, or β-irradiation is indicated.

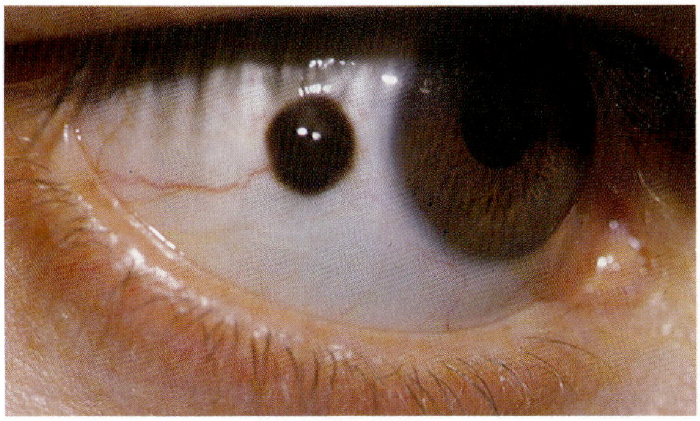

Fig. 2.6.3 Conjunctival naevus.

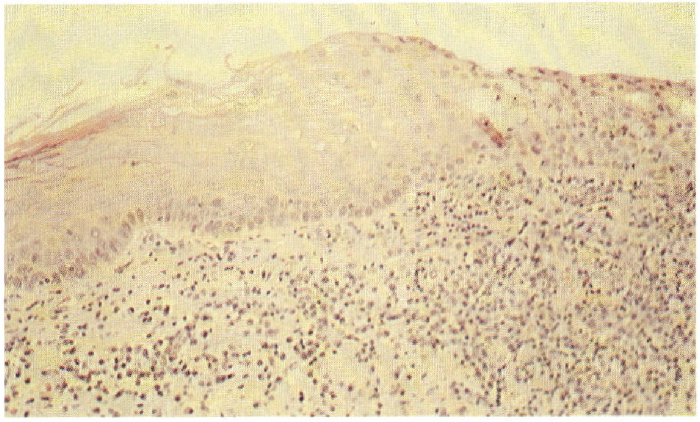

Fig. 2.6.6 Histological section showing squamous metaplasia of the conjunctiva (haematoxylin and eosin stain).

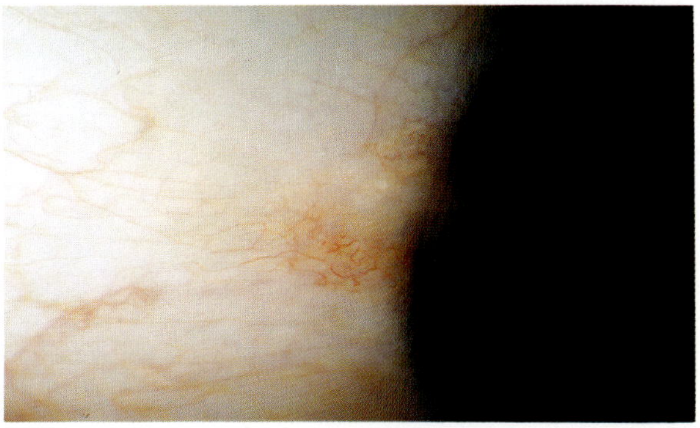

Fig. 2.6.4 Cystic naevus of the conjunctiva.

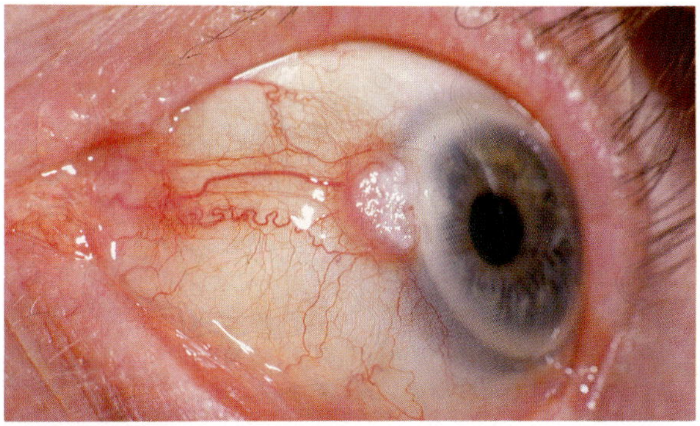

Fig. 2.6.7 Conjunctival carcinoma in situ.

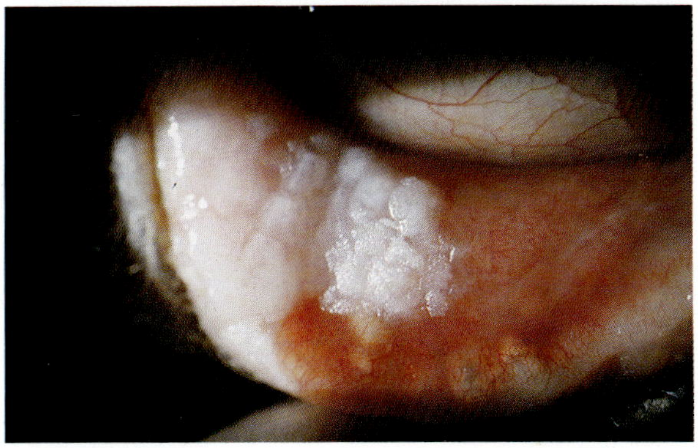

Fig. 2.6.5 Squamous metaplasia of the conjunctiva.

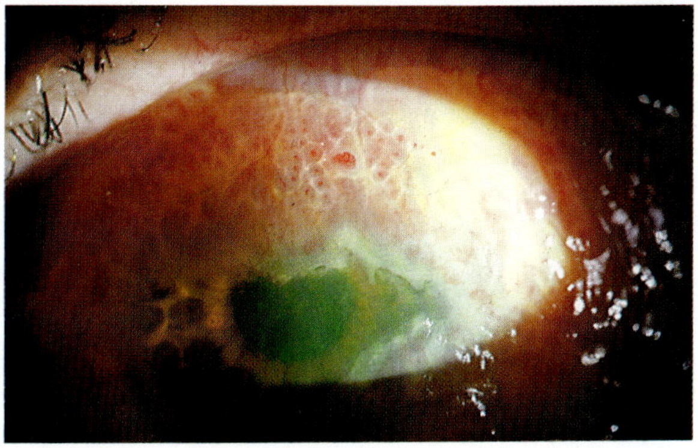

Fig. 2.6.8 Squamous cell carcinoma of the conjunctiva.

Lymphoma (Fig. 2.6.9)

Conjunctival lymphoma may be the first manifestation of systemic disease. The lesion characteristically presents as a diffuse pinkish infiltrate. Biopsy confirms the diagnosis. Care should be taken in biopsying lesions in the upper outer aspect in case the lacrimal gland or its ducts be damaged. Treatment depends on the type of tumour and the extent of spread. If the disease is localized to the conjunctiva, local irradiation is effective.

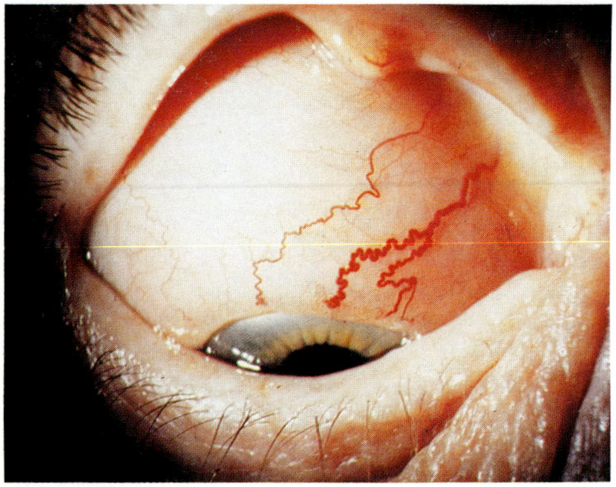

Fig. 2.6.9 Conjunctival lymphoma.

Melanoma (Fig. 2.6.10)

Melanoma of the conjunctiva is rare, and, like melanomas in other sites, its behaviour is unpredictable. Fifteen per cent of patients die from systemic metastases within five years of diagnosis, large tumours greater than 2 mm in depth having a particularly poor prognosis. The tumour may arise de novo, in an area of acquired melanosis, or from a pre-existing naevus. It may be difficult to distinguish from a naevus, and in cases of doubt, biopsy should be undertaken. Full examination should be undertaken to assess the extent of any local or distant spread. Localized melanomas should be excised completely, using frozen section control, and the surrounding area should be treated with double freeze-thaw cryotherapy. The response to radiotherapy is variable.

Recurrent or very extensive lesions infiltrating the orbit or globe require exenteration.

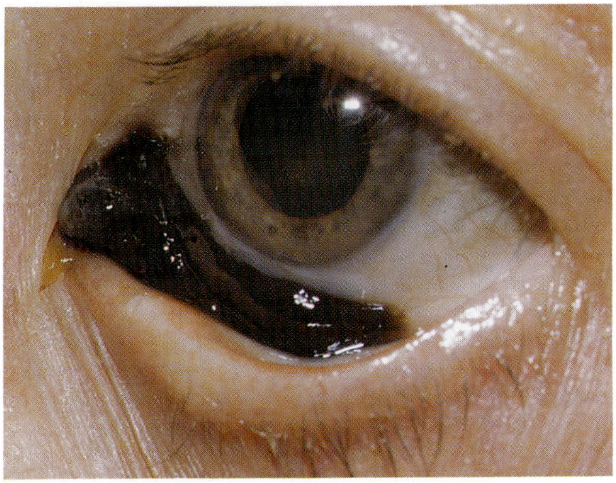

Fig. 2.6.10 Malignant melanoma involving both palpebral and bulbar conjunctiva.

DEPOSITIONS

Argyrosis (Fig. 2.7.1)

Depositions of reduced silver are seen in the conjunctiva following chronic exposure to silver. Now uncommon, the condition was seen frequently when silver nitrate was used as a disinfectant and in nasal drops. The deposition is commonly seen in silversmiths.

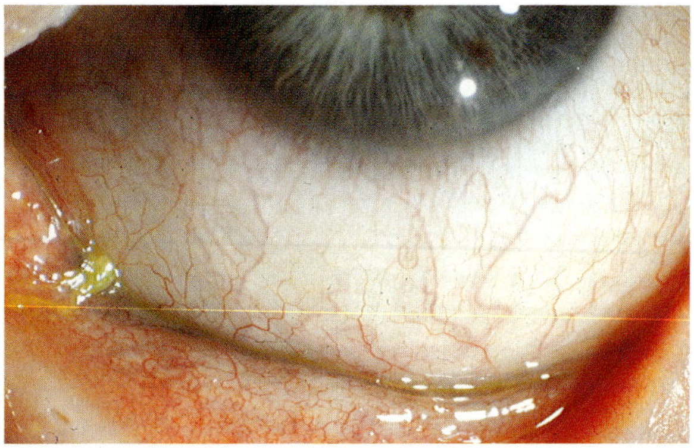

Fig. 2.7.1 Argyrosis of the conjunctiva.

Alkaptonuria

This metabolic disorder is inherited in an autosomal recessive manner. A deficiency in the enzyme homogentisic acid oxidase leads to a generalized deposition of pigment in connective tissue; this is termed 'ochronosis'. The sclera and ears (Fig. 2.7.2) are first affected, but later in the disease the conjunctiva becomes discolored also (Fig. 2.7.3). An associated arthritis is characterized by acute inflammatory episodes, and eventually ankylosis of the lumbo-sacral spine.

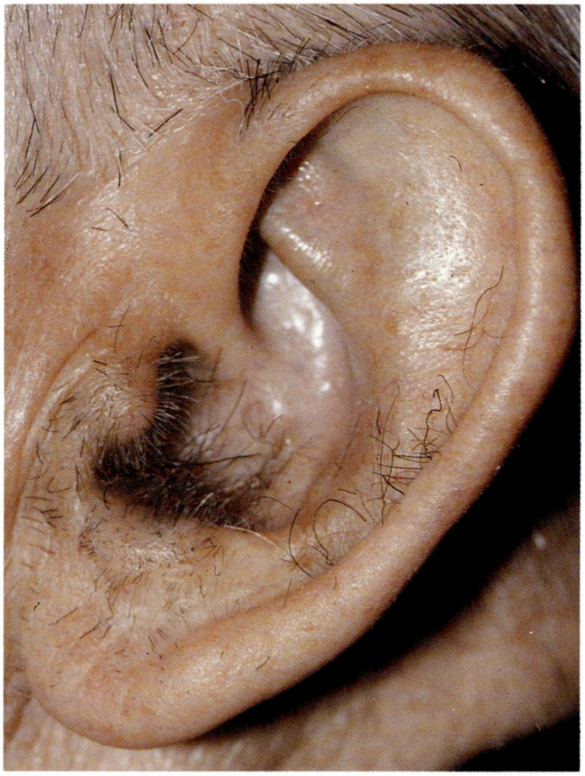

Fig. 2.7.2 Ochronosis showing pigmentation of the earlobes.

Jaundice (Fig. 2.7.4)

In jaundice there is a widespread deposition of bilirubin and, to a lesser extent, biliverdin in the tissues. It is usually first apparent in the sclera once the plasma bilirubin exceeds 50 μmol/l (normal 5–17 umol/l). The conjunctiva is involved later in the disease. Normalization of serum bilirubin levels is followed by fading of the conjunctival pigmentation.

Drugs

Chronic use of topical adrenaline leads to deposition of adrenochrome deposits in the conjunctiva (Fig. 2.7.5). The phenomenon has also been noted, though more rarely, with the adrenaline pro-drug dipivefrin. Systemic drugs commonly causing conjunctival discoloration include chlorpromazine, which produces a golden-brown colour, and gold, used in the treatment of rheumatoid arthritis (chrysiasis).

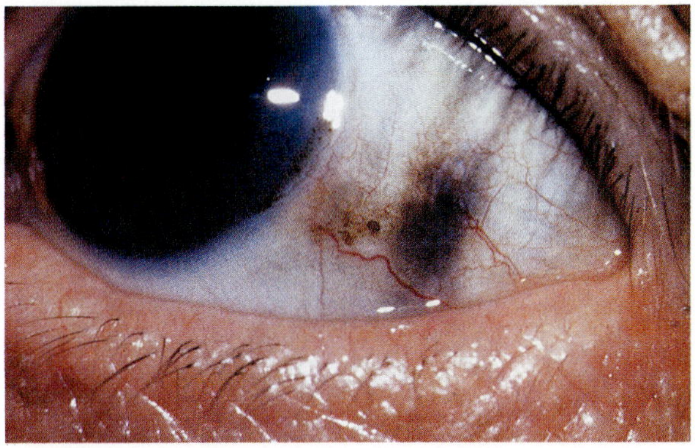

Fig. 2.7.3 Conjunctival and scleral pigmentation in ochronosis.

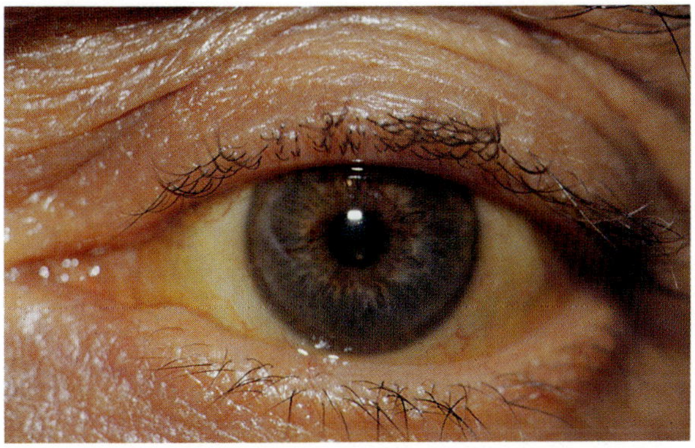

Fig. 2.7.4 Conjunctival pigmentation in jaundice.

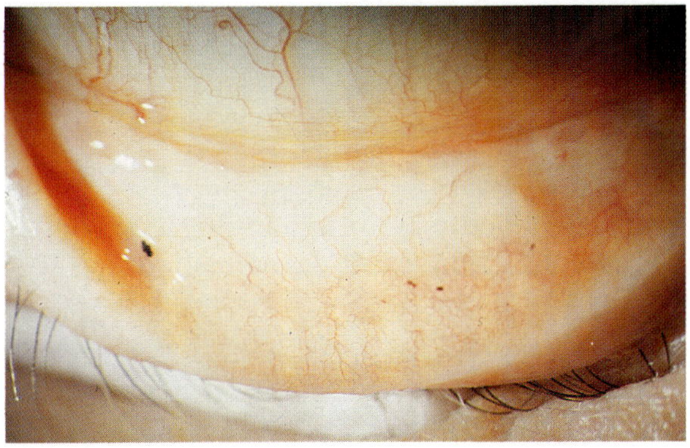

Fig. 2.7.5 Adrenochrome deposits in the conjunctiva following topical adrenaline therapy.

ALLERGIC EYE DISEASE

Allergic conjunctivitis

This has several manifestations, but all are caused by allergen binding to cell-bound IgE, leading to eosinophil and mast cell degranulation.

Acute chemosis (Fig. 2.8.1)

This can result from sensitization to many topical allergens. Itching is marked and the conjunctival oedema may be extreme. The condition subsides quickly once exposure to the allergen is restricted.

Papillary conjunctivitis (Fig. 2.8.2)

Seasonal and perennial papillary conjunctivitis are more chronic disorders often found in atopic individuals. The allergen may be difficult to identify, and treatment is based upon prophylaxis with topical cromoglycate and symptomatic relief with cold compresses and topical antihistamines and vasoconstrictors.

The diagnosis is based upon the history and the presence of other atopic disorders (asthma, eczema, perennial rhinitis) in the patient or family. Serum IgE levels are often raised, and conjunctival scrapes or biopsy show large numbers of eosinophils.

Vernal conjunctivitis

This usually develops in atopic individuals during their second decade. Symptoms vary from mild to debilitating, with itching, tearing, photophobia and thick stringy mucoid discharge.

Limbal vernal (Fig. 2.8.3)

This is characterized by a broad thickened limbus, with elevations which typically appear gelatinous. Small white lesions composed of collections of eosinophils occur, termed Horner–Tranta dots.

Palpebral vernal (Fig. 2.8.4)

This is manifest by a chronic papillary conjunctivitis, often displaying large 'cobblestone' papillae under the upper lid.

Keratitis

Both limbal and palpebral disease can be complicated by a keratitis which consists of a superficial punctate keratopathy in its earliest form, but which may progress to ulceration. This is typically shield-shaped, but may appear as a plaque (Fig. 2.8.5) which resolves to leave a superficial scar (Fig. 2.8.6).

Treatment

Treatment for mild disease is symptomatic, and rests upon the use of cromoglycate and antihistamines. When symptoms are more marked, or when keratitis is present, topical steroid is required. Because of the chronicity of this disease and the disordered immune response in these patients, steroid use is particularly prone to side-effects such as herpetic infection, cataract formation and glaucoma.

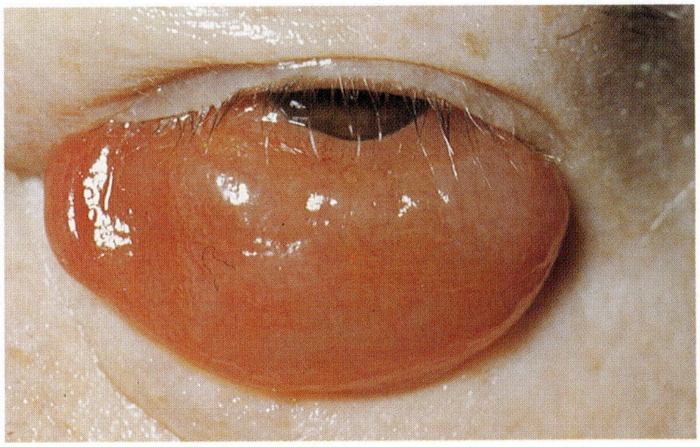

Fig. 2.8.1 Acute chemosis.

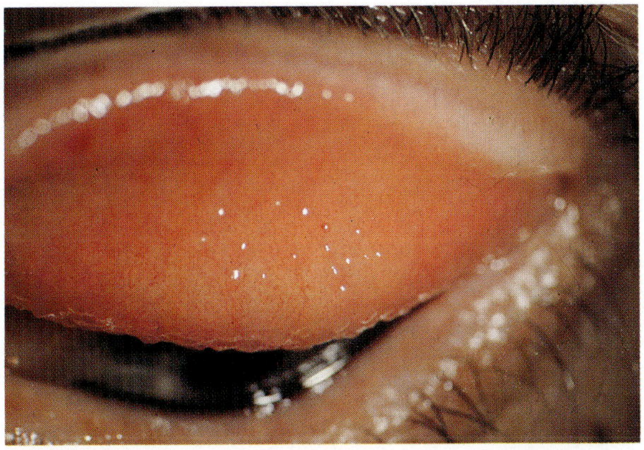

Fig. 2.8.2 Chronic allergic papillary conjunctivitis.

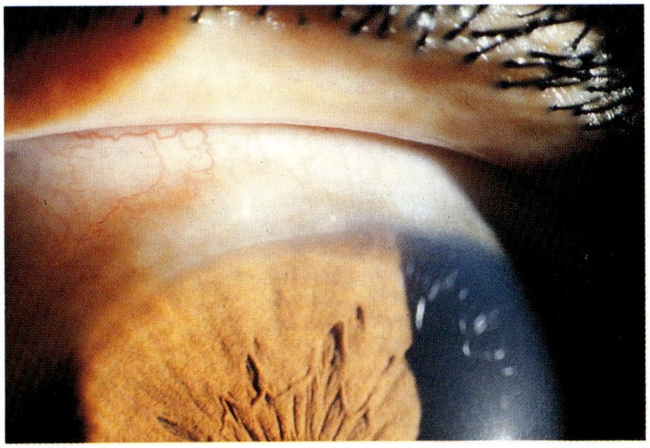

Fig. 2.8.3 Limbal vernal conjunctivitis demonstrating Horner–Tranta dots.

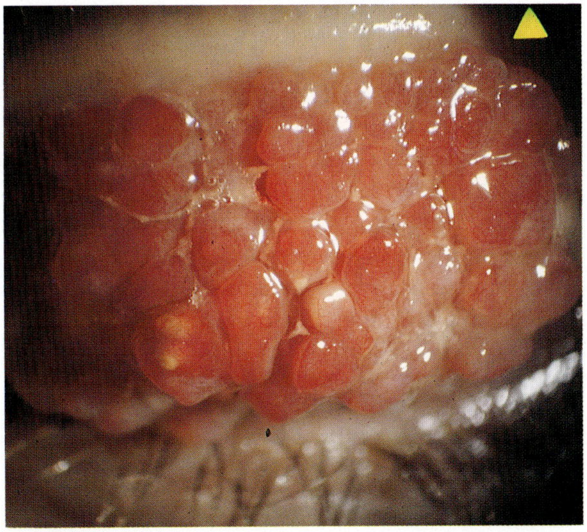

Fig. 2.8.4 Cobblestone papillae in vernal conjunctivitis.

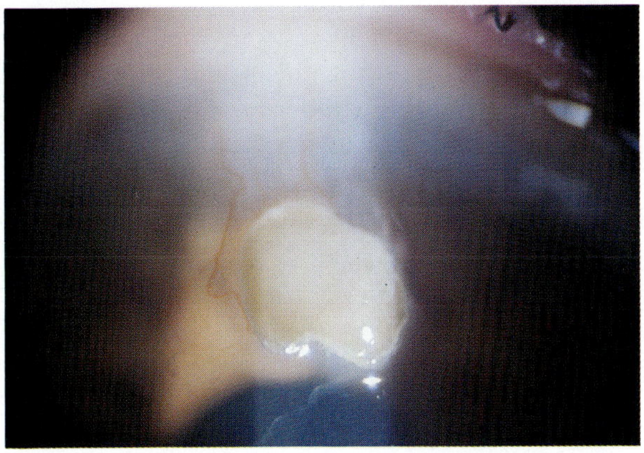

Fig. 2.8.5 Corneal plaque in vernal conjunctivitis.

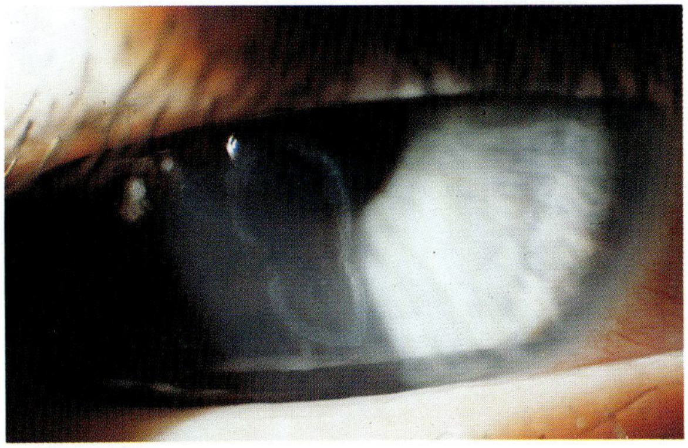

Fig. 2.8.6 Superficial corneal scarring following vernal conjunctivitis.

Atopic keratoconjunctivitis (Fig. 2.8.7)

Atopic adults may develop a chronic keratoconjunctivitis characterized by papillary conjunctivitis, blepharitis, chemosis and a chronic punctate keratitis with vascularization and scarring. Symptoms are similar to those of vernal disease, with itching, burning, lacrimation and photophobia.

Keratoconus, typical shield-shaped cataracts, and herpes simplex keratitis are associated features. Management should be as for vernal disease.

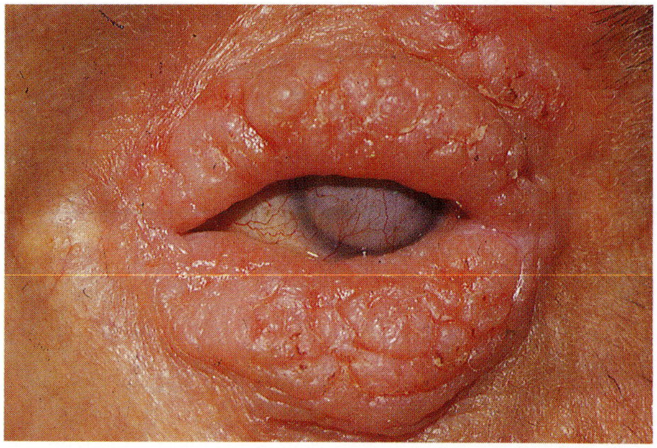

Fig. 2.8.7 Keratoconjunctivitis with marked lid thickening and corneal vascularization.

Giant papillary conjunctivitis (Fig. 2.8.8)

This is a chronic conjunctivitis characterized by large tarsal papillae, which can develop following contact lens wear or chronic irritation from an orbital prosthesis or sutures.

Treatment should include meticulous lens or prosthesis hygiene together with the use of preservative-free preparations and cromoglycate. Sometimes a change in material of contact lens or prosthesis is required.

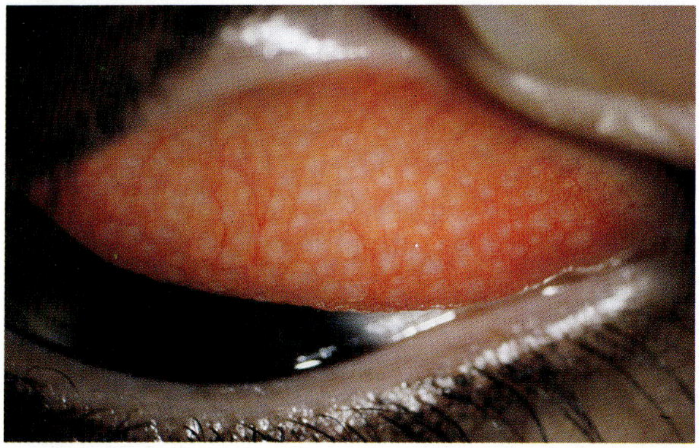

Fig. 2.8.8 Giant papillary conjunctivitis following contact lens wear.

Contact dermatitis (Fig. 2.8.9)

A number of topically applied drugs can produce a periocular skin eruption due to a type IV delayed hypersensitivity response. Atropine and neomycin are particularly prone to excite such a response, although most agents can in susceptible individuals. Treatment is the withdrawal of the drug.

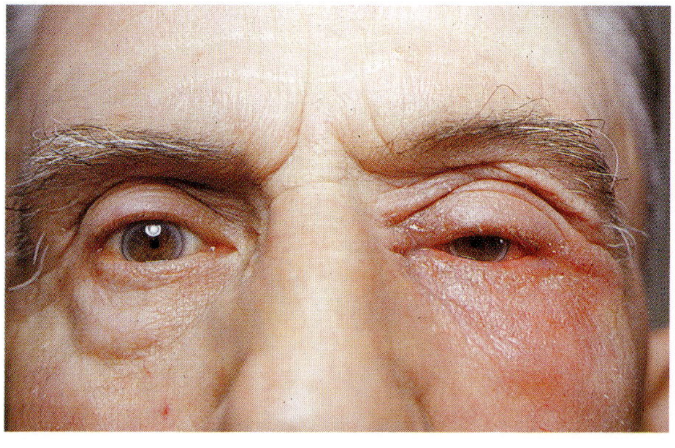

Fig. 2.8.9 Contact dermatitis following topical antibiotic treatment.

FURTHER READING

Anatomy

Wolff E 1976 Anatomy of the eye and orbit, 7th edition revised by R Warwick. H K Lewis, London

Conjunctivitis

Rapoza P A, Quinn T C, Terry A C 1990 A systematic approach to the diagnosis and treatment of chronic conjunctivitis. American Journal of Ophthalmology 109: 138–142

Tabbara K F, Hyndiuk R A (eds) 1986 Infections of the eye. Little Brown, Boston

Ullman S, Roussel T J Forster R K 1987 Gonococcal keratoconjunctivitis. Survey of Ophthalmology 32: 199–208

The dry eye

Smolin G, Friedlaender M H (eds) 1988 Management of the dry eye. International Ophthalmology Clinics 28.

Cicatricial conjunctivitis

Foster C S 1986 Cicatricial pemphigoid. Transactions of the American Ophthalmologic Society 84: 527–663

Lightman S 1989 Bullous disorders of the skin affecting the conjunctiva. In: Lightman S (ed) Immunology of eye diseases. Kluwer, Dordrecht, p 9–21

Sandford-Smith J 1986 Eye diseases in hot climates. Wright, Bristol

Wright P 1986 Cicatrizing conjunctivitis. Transactions of the Ophthalmological Society of the United Kingdom 105: 1–17

Benign conjunctival lesions

Harkey M E, Metz H S 1968 Cryotherapy of conjunctival papillomata. American Journal of Ophthalmology 66: 872–874

Jaros P A, DeLuise V P 1988 Pingueculae and pterygia. Survey of Ophthalmology 33: 41–49

Spaide R F, Ward D L 1990 Conjunctival biopsy in the diagnosis of sarcoidosis. British Journal of Ophthalmology 74: 469–471

Premalignant and malignant lesions

Jakobiec F A, Iwamoto T, Patell M, Knowles D M II 1986 Ocular adnexal monoclonal lymphoid tumors with a favorable prognosis. Ophthalmology 93: 47–57

Jakobiec F A, Rini F J, Fraunfelder F T, Brownstein S 1988 Cryotherapy for conjunctival primary acquired melanosis and malignant melanoma. Experience with 62 cases. Ophthalmology 95: 1058–1070

Conjunctival depositions

Scriver C R, Beaudet A L, Sly W S, Valle D (eds) 1989 The metabolic basis of inherited disease. McGraw Hill, New York

Allergic disease

Foster C S 1988 The Cromolyn sodium collaborative study group. Evaluation of topical cromolyn sodium in the treatment of vernal keratoconjunctivitis. Ophthalmology 95: 194–201

Smolin G, Friedlaender M H (eds) 1988 Ocular allergy. International Ophthalmology Clinics 28

3
THE CORNEA

ANATOMY

The cornea consists of five layers which are the epithelium and its basement membrane, Bowman's membrane, the stroma, Descemet's membrane and the endothelium (Fig. 3.1.1). All layers are ectodermal in origin, the epithelium being derived from epidermal ectoderm, and all other layers from neural crest cells. Failure of normal migration of ectodermal cells is responsible for the 'neurocristopathies' which manifest as a number of endothelial, iris and angle anomalies.

The epithelium consists of five or six layers of cells, the innermost of which are columnar, and the outermost squamous, with a gradual transition between these cell types through the other layers. Microvilli project from the outer cell membranes of the squamous cell layer. The innermost layer is connected to the underlying basement membrane by hemidesmosomes.

Beneath the epithelium lies Bowman's membrane, which is acellular and collagenous. The stroma lies deep to this, and constitutes 90% of the thickness of the cornea. It is made up of keratocytes and lamellae of collagen fibrils arranged in a regular 64 nm banding pattern. Maintenance of its clarity depends on dehydration which is achieved through active metabolic activity in the endothelium.

The endothelium is the innermost layer, and secretes Descemet's membrane, which lies between it and the stroma. The endothelium is a monolayer of cells which cannot be regenerated. At birth the density of cells is up to 7500 cells/mm^2 but this rapidly declines to about 2500 cells/mm^2 in the adult. The cells are hexagonal in shape, with oligocilia present on some. The cells are separated by a 30 μm gap, with tight junctions at the apical part of the cell (Fig. 3.1.2).

The cornea is supplied by branches of the anterior ciliary nerves and the conjunctival nerves, which form a pericorneal plexus. Sixty to eighty myelinated trunks pass radially into the cornea, 2 to 4 mm into which they lose their myelin and divide. An intraepithelial and a subepithelial plexus of nerves are formed, as well as a stromal plexus. All layers of the cornea except Descemet's membrane have a rich nerve supply.

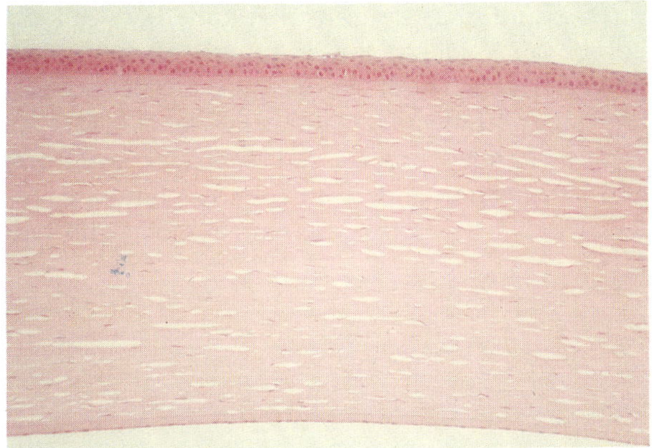

Fig. 3.1.1 Histological section of the normal cornea (haematoxylin and eosin stain).

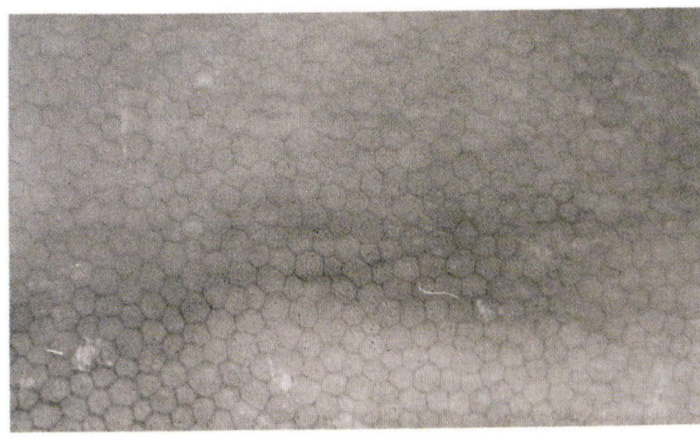

Fig. 3.1.2 Specular microscopy of the corneal endothelium showing hexagonal cells (courtesy of Mr A. Patterson).

The limbus is the transition zone between the cornea and sclera, and is populated by multi-potential cells, both on its outer (conjunctival) and inner (trabecular) surfaces (Fig. 3.1.3).

The normal cornea is an avascular structure, and its nutrition is derived from the limbal capillaries and lymphatics, the aqueous and the tear film.

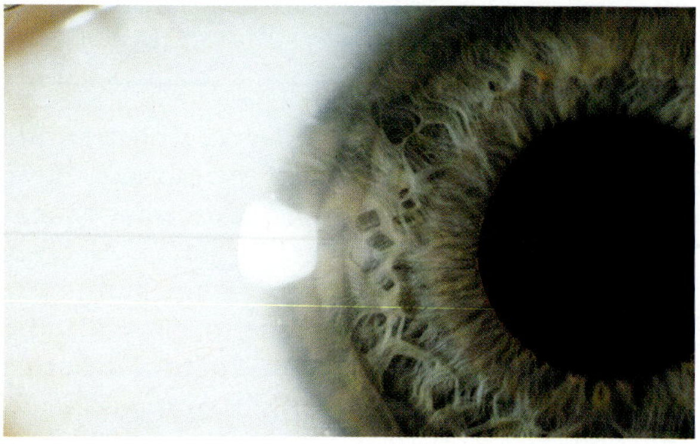

Fig. 3.1.3 The limbus.

VIRAL KERATITIS

Herpes simplex

Herpes simplex virus (HSV) infection is the commonest cause of corneal opacity in the Western world, and up to 80% of the population have antibodies to the virus. Two serotypes exist: type 1 and type 2. The former is by far the more common, and HSV type 2 rarely causes ocular disease.

The ocular manifestations of HSV type 1 infection are variable, and dependent on previous infection, the immune status of the patient, coexisting eye disease and current and past treatment.

The infection can affect all layers of the cornea, and may be transient with complete resolution, or lead to severe chronic disease. Recognition of different disease patterns in the cornea is important in the development of an effective management plan.

Dendritic ulcer

The characteristic branching 'dendritic ulcer' of the corneal epithelium is seen in both primary HSV infection of a host with no prior immunity and in recurrent disease in which latent virus is reactivated. It stains readily with both fluorescein (Fig. 3.2.1), which stains the base of the ulcer, and Rose Bengal (Fig. 3.2.2), which stains the edges. The epithelial defect is not always dendritic in form, and punctate epithelial keratitis and small areas of heaped epithelium are commonly seen.

Primary infection is often associated also with a vesicular eruption (Fig. 3.2.3) of the eyelid skin, but these lesions may be small and easily missed. An associated follicular or pseudomembranous conjunctivitis and regional lympadenopathy are common. Uveitis may also accompany a primary infection.

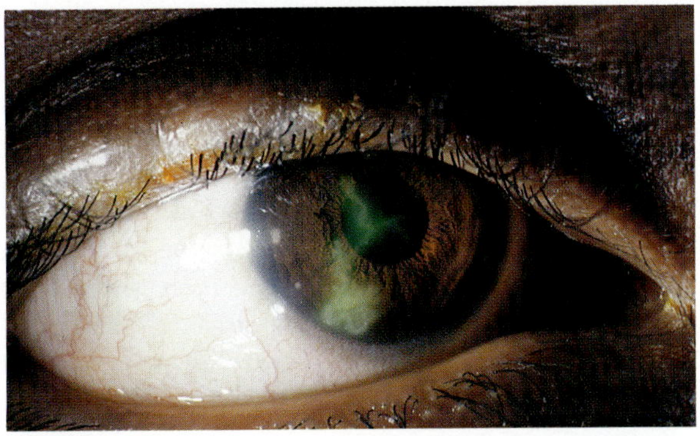

Fig. 3.2.1 Dendritic ulcer stained with fluorescein.

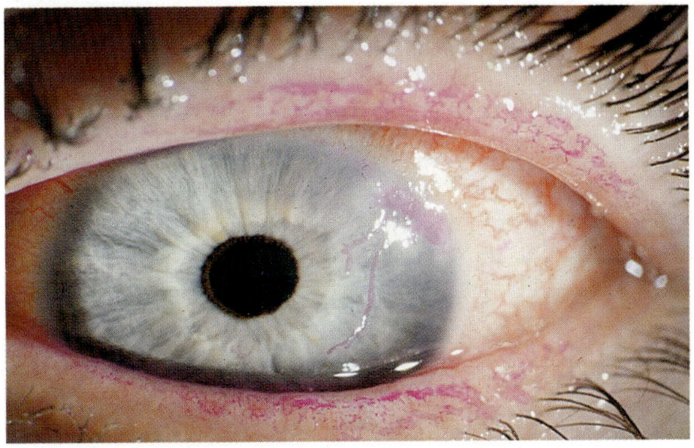

Fig. 3.2.2 Dendritic ulcer stained with Rose Bengal.

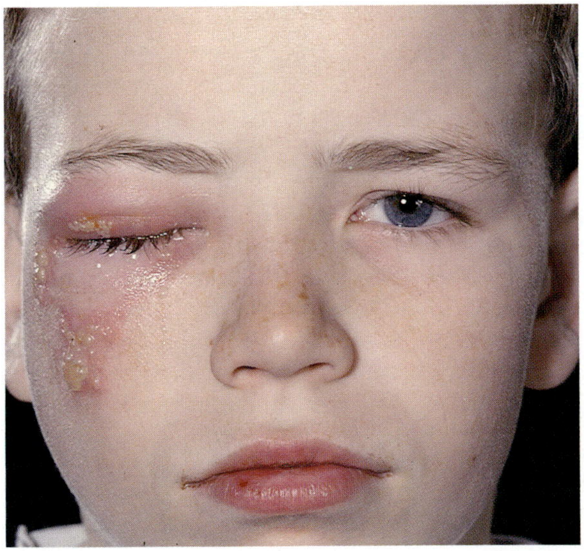

Fig. 3.2.3 Vesicular skin eruption in primary herpes simplex infection.

HSV infection of atopic subjects can be particularly virulent. Kaposi's varicelliform eruption (Fig. 3.2.4) occurs when eczematous skin becomes infected with HSV and can be life threatening in small children.

Dendritic ulcers normally respond well to the administration of topical antivirals. Acyclovir, which is activated by HSV-induced thymidine kinase, has the advantage of low toxicity, in contrast to some of the earlier agents. A two-week course of acyclovir five times daily is usually effective.

Amoebic ulcer

This develops from a dendritic ulcer if corticosteroid is used. The area of ulceration adopts an amoeboid or 'geographic' configuration, and represents rapid proliferation of the virus in the face of local immunosuppression. The lesion stains strikingly with fluorescein (Fig. 3.2.5). The stroma may subsequently become invaded by virus also, and if steroid treatment is maintained, lead to perforation. Treatment should be the staged withdrawal of steroid, and institution of topical antiviral therapy.

Pseudodendrites (Fig. 3.2.6)

These are epithelial lesions composed of mucus deposits which adopt a dendritic pattern, but, in contrast to true dendritic ulcers, they do not represent active viral replication. As well as occurring in HSV infection, they are seen also in herpes zoster infection and in tear film deficiency states. The term 'mucous plaque' is also used to describe these deposits, which may also occur in a more diffuse configuration.

Treatment should include administration of tear film substitutes and mucolytics, such as acetylcysteine. Debridement of the cornea is necessary if these measures alone are not sufficient.

Metaherpetic ulceration (Fig. 3.2.7)

This is a chronic indolent ulceration which persists beyond the period of active viral replication. It is typically ovoid in shape, with a smooth, heaped margin, and stains poorly, if at all. Damage to the basement membrane of the epithelium, together with toxicity of antivirals, contribute to its chronicity. Corneal sensation is often reduced or absent.

Metaherpetic keratitis may progress to lysis of the stroma, and perforation. Treatment should include optimization of corneal environment, by treating any coexisting lid disease and providing tear supplements if necessary, as well as reducing topical steroid treatment as much as possible. Antivirals used should be non-toxic to the epithelium.

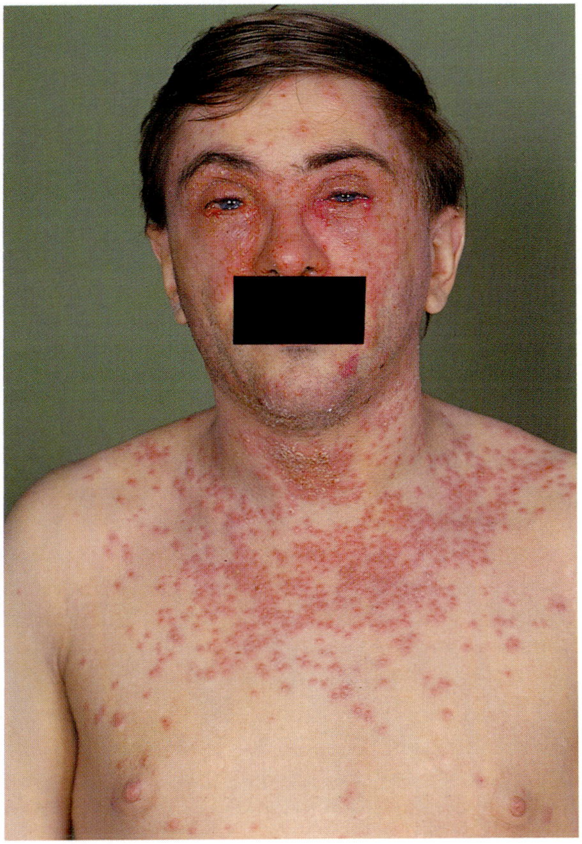

Fig. 3.2.4 Kaposi's varicelliform eruption (eczema herpeticum) (courtesy of Department of Dermatology, Royal Hallamshire Hospital).

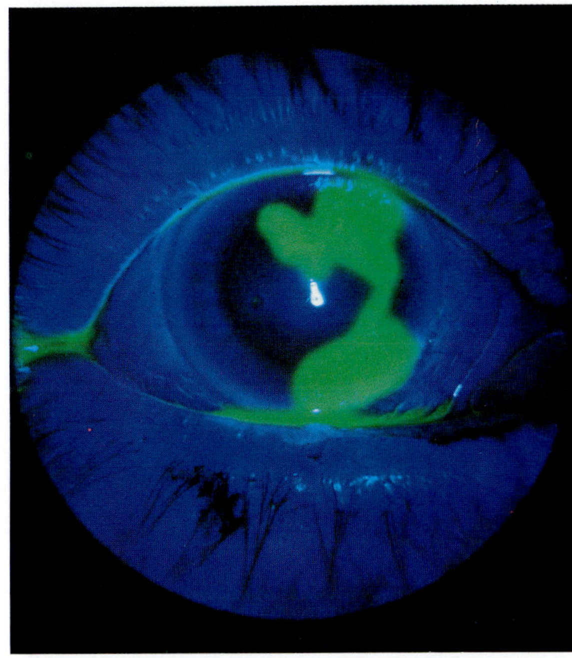

Fig. 3.2.5 Amoebic ulcer stained with fluorescein and viewed in blue light (courtesy of Mr C. A. L. Palmer).

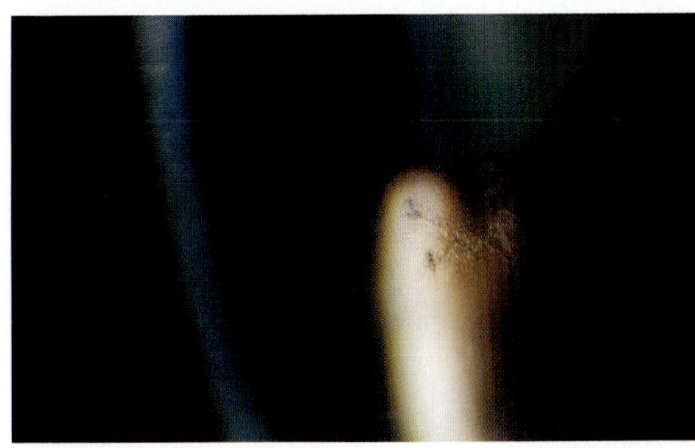

Fig. 3.2.6 Pseudodendrites.

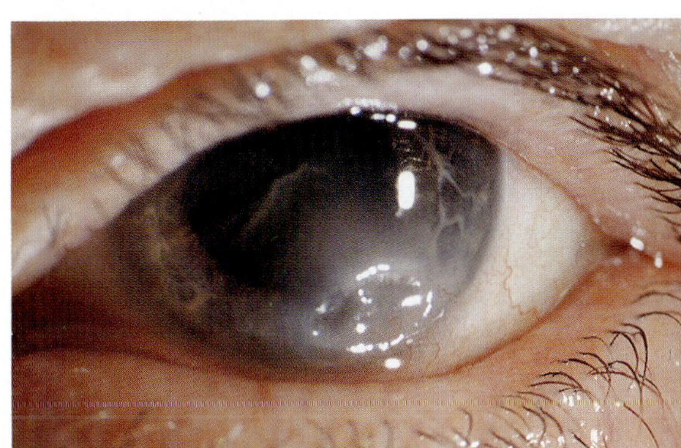

Fig. 3.2.7 Metaherpetic ulceration of the cornea.

Stromal disease (Fig. 3.2.8)

Although a mild stromal oedema may accompany the epithelial lesion of primary HSV infection, a severe stromal inflammatory reaction is a feature of recurrent disease. It represents primarily a delayed hypersensitivity reaction to the HSV antigen, although secondary bacterial infection or continued HSV replication may contribute to it.

The classical 'disciform keratitis' (Fig. 3.2.9) consists of a central or paracentral stromal oedema, often associated with a uveitis, and responds well to low-dose topical steroid given with topical antiviral cover to prevent reactivation of the HSV.

Other patterns of stromal disease are seen and include focal infiltrates and the 'immune ring', which represents immune complex deposition.

Stromal disease is often recurrent, and the resultant scarring can seriously compromise vision, necessitating keratoplasty (Fig. 3.2.10). Recurrent disease following corneal grafting is common.

Varicella zoster

The varicella zoster virus, like HSV, can affect the eye either as a primary infection in a previously unexposed host (varicella or chickenpox), or by reactivation of latent virus remaining in sensory ganglia following previous infection (zoster).

Corneal involvement in chickenpox is unusual, but it can lead to a mild punctate keratitis, marginal ulceration, disciform reaction and even corneal lysis.

Herpes zoster is far more commonly associated with corneal disease, presenting a variety of appearances.

Skin eruption (Fig. 3.2.11)

The dermatome distribution of the skin eruption associated with zoster reflects the reactivation of quiescent virus stored in sensory ganglia. In herpes zoster ophthalmicus (HZO) the first division of the trigeminal nerve is affected, although concomitant involvement of the second (maxillary) branch is not uncommon. Hutchinson's sign of vesicular eruption of the skin on the side of the tip or the side of the mid-portion of the nose indicates a high chance of ocular involvement, and such patients should be followed closely. Corneal sensation may be lost early in the disease, and be associated with persistent corneal pathology.

Pain and paraesthesia precede the vesicular skin eruptions, which normally last three weeks. Severe scarring and post-herpetic neuralgia may persist for years, however, and be recalcitrant to treatment.

Dendritic ulcer

Active replication of herpes zoster virus within the corneal epithelium may manifest as a dendritic ulcer. In contrast to dendrites seen in HSV infection, those seen with zoster tend to be small, often multiple, and poorly staining. Other epithelial defects range from mild punctate keratitis to extensive ulceration. Loss of corneal sensation and cicatricial distortion of the lids and lash position may perpetuate epithelial disease, and secondary bacterial infection may supervene.

The role of antivirals in the management of zoster infection is controversial, but a short course of a non-epithelial toxic topical preparation at the time of the appearance of dendrites is probably beneficial.

Nummular keratitis (Fig. 3.2.12)

This is a superficial stromal response, characterized by numerous small, irregular, whitish patches which follow herpes zoster ophthalmicus. The lesions do not stain, and they rarely interfere with visual acuity, but if they do, topical steroid usually leads to resolution. Unfortunately, cessation of treatment is often followed by recurrence.

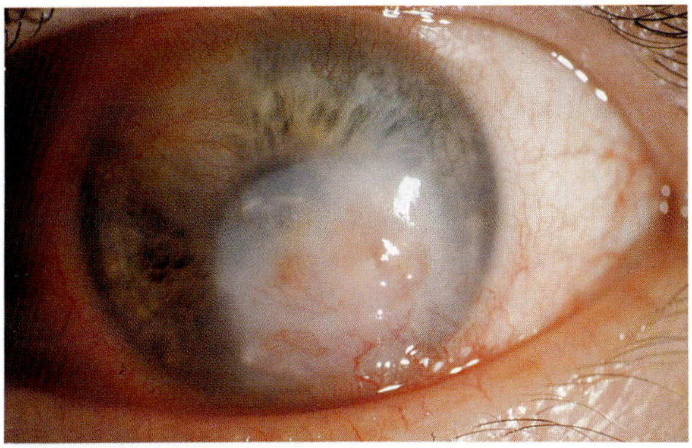

Fig. 3.2.8 Stromal disease due to active herpes simplex virus replication.

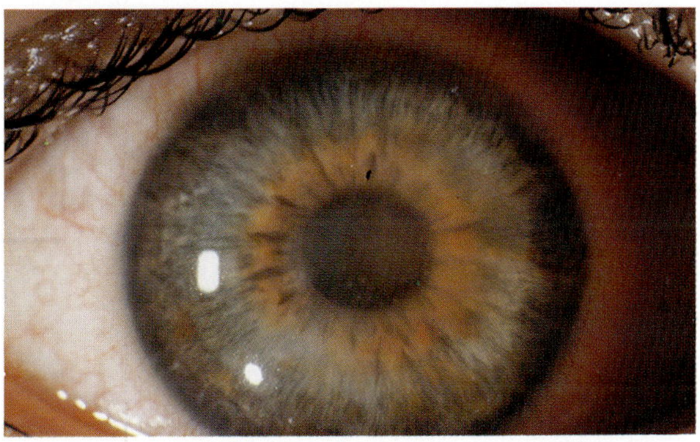

Fig. 3.2.9 Disciform keratitis.

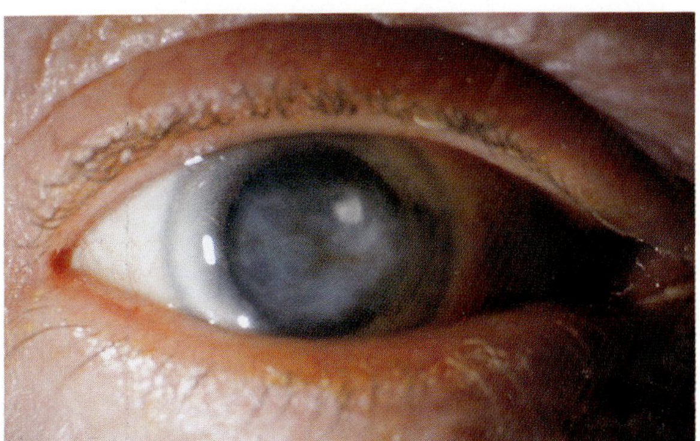

Fig. 3.2.10 Stromal scarring following herpes simplex infection.

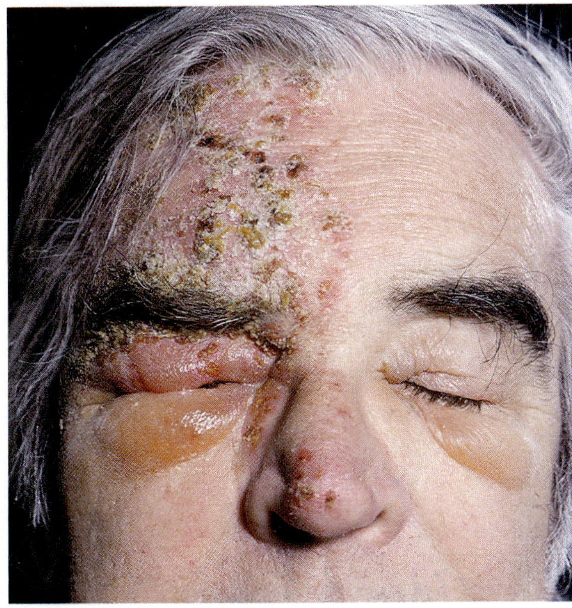

Fig. 3.2.11 Vesicular skin eruption in herpes zoster infection. Note involvement of skin of the tip of the nose (Hutchinson's sign).

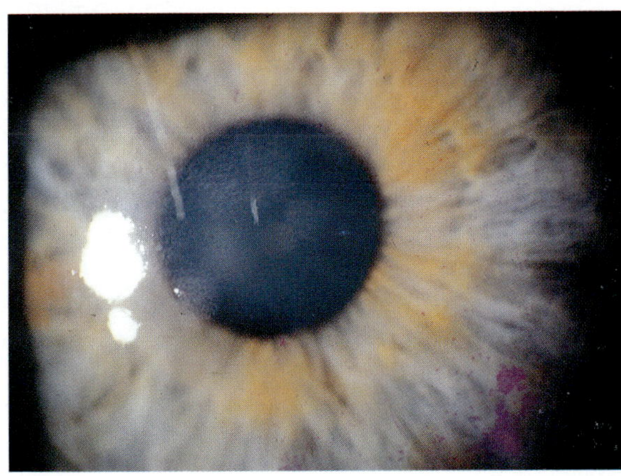

Fig. 3.2.12 Nummular keratitis.

Disciform keratitis

This is an immune-mediated stromal response to reactivation of the varicella zoster virus, which is often chronic. Treatment is with topical antivirals. Topical steroids may be used in addition, but these may prolong the course of the disease, and recurrence is common on their withdrawal. Care must be taken if there is corneal thinning not to induce perforation.

Stromal scarring is often the end result, together with vascular ingrowth and cholesterol deposition (Fig. 3.2.13), and requires penetrating keratoplasty. Such corneal grafts are prone to recurrent zoster, and, if the cornea is vascularized, to an increased incidence of allograft rejection.

Mucous plaque keratitis (Fig. 3.2.14)

This indolent ulceration may present a variety of patterns. Pseudodendrites of heaped-up epithelial and mucous cells may form, or there may be more diffuse ulcerated areas. The condition requires similar management to the chronic metaherpetic ulceration seen in HSV infection, but whereas corticosteroids are contraindicated in HSV epithelial disease they may be of benefit in zoster-mediated ulceration.

Adenovirus

Adenovirus infection of the eye usually leads to an acute self-resolving follicular conjunctivitis. Epidemic keratoconjunctivitis is seen with serotypes 5, 8, 10 and 19, as well as with certain intermediate serotypes.

When the cornea is involved a transient superficial punctate keratitis usually occurs, but in some cases sub-epithelial infiltrates develop (Fig. 3.2.15) which can persist and affect visual acuity. Although topical steroid reduces their incidence, and also aids their resolution, recurrence is common on withdrawal of therapy.

Adenovirus infection rarely produces an acute stromal oedema, and consequent scarring may necessitate keratoplasty.

Thygeson's keratitis (Fig. 3.2.16)

This is a keratitis of presumed viral origin which is characterized by subepithelial infiltrates and superficial punctate keratitis, in the absence of lid or conjunctival inflammation. The infiltrates usually resolve spontaneously but are prone to recurrence. Their resolution can be hastened by the application of topical corticosteroids.

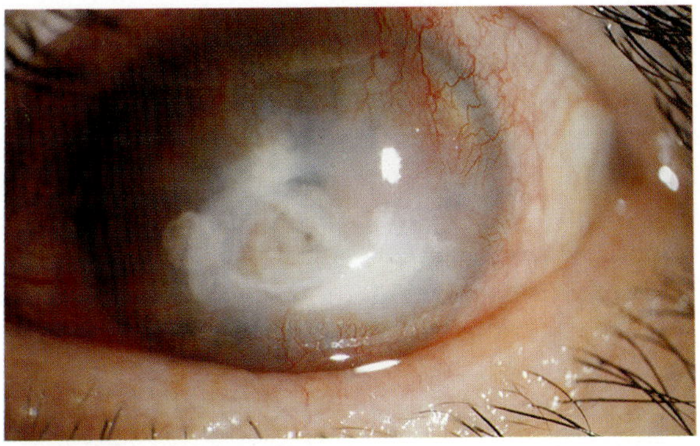

Fig. 3.2.13 Stromal scarring and thinning and vascularization in herpes zoster.

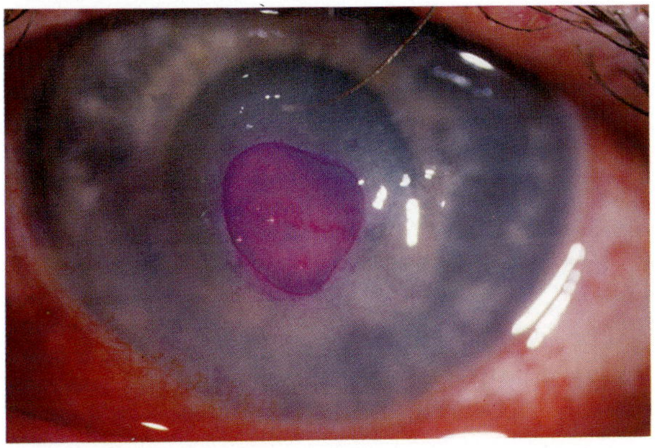

Fig. 3.2.14 Mucous plaque keratitis stained with Rose Bengal.

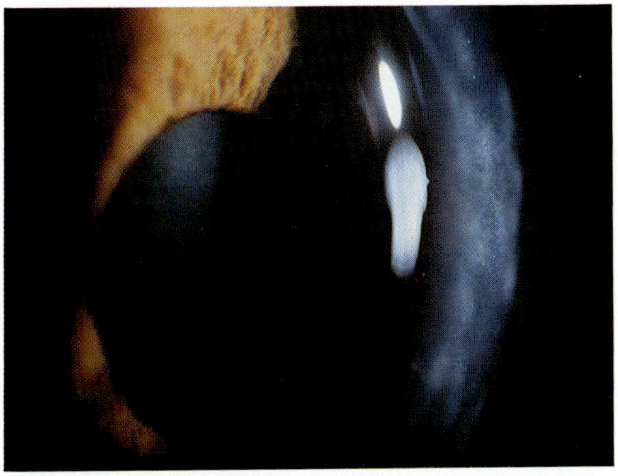

Fig. 3.2.15 Subepithelial corneal infiltrates associated with adenovirus infection.

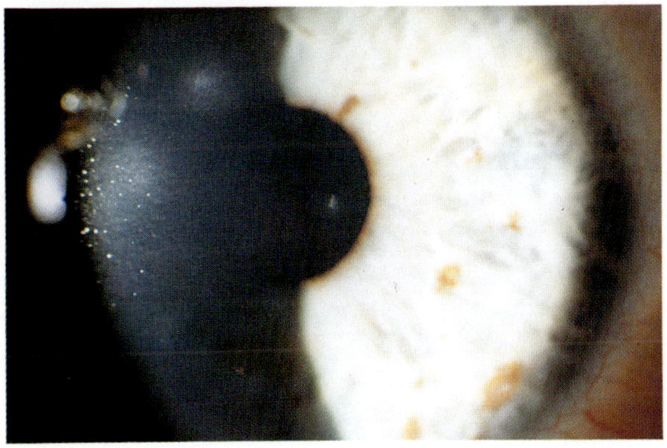

Fig. 3.2.16 Thygeson's keratitis with small subepithelial infiltrates.

INFECTIVE NON-VIRAL KERATITIS

Bacterial keratitis (Fig. 3.3.1)

Bacterial keratitis causes pain, loss of vision, redness, swelling and a conjunctival discharge. A central corneal ulcer is usually present, and often an associated hypopyon. Several organisms can be responsible for this clinical picture, and full microbiological investigation must be initiated prior to antibiotic treatment.

Contact lens wear, trauma, corneal oedema, keratoconjunctivitis sicca, herpes simplex infection and drug therapy all predispose to infection.

The commonest bacterial pathogens include pseudomonas spp., staphylococcus spp., streptococcus spp. and enterobacteria.

Since progressive corneal destruction can be rapid, antibiotic therapy must be started before the organism has been identified and drug sensitivity established. Frequent topical strong antibiotics are recommended as indicated by a gram stain of the corneal scrape. If no organism is detected, then treatment with broad-spectrum antibiotics is indicated.

Fungal keratitis (Fig. 3.3.2)

Keratitis produced by invasive fungi is becoming more frequent. The presentation may be less dramatic than that of bacterial keratitis and be resistant to antibiotic therapy. Fungi should be sought in the microbiological work-up of all patients with ulcerative keratitis.

Fusarium sp. and aspergillus sp. are the most frequent pathogens, but many other fungal species have been reported to cause keratitis.

Antifungal agents available include amphotericin B, natamycin and newer agents such as ketaconazole and flucytosine.

Acanthamoeba (Fig. 3.3.3)

Acanthamoeba is recognized as an ocular pathogen with increasing frequency, particularly in contact lens wearers who use contaminated lens cleaning solutions.

The condition is frequently misdiagnosed as viral or bacterial keratitis initially, and the poor prognosis often associated with acanthamoeba keratitis is in part due to a delay in diagnosis.

Cardinal features are a stromal keratitis, often appearing as a ring infiltrate, with satellite lesions and a radial keratoneuritis. Progression to the limbus and sclera can occur, as can corneal thinning, descemetocoele formation and perforation.

Diagnosis is dependent upon identification of the acanthamoeba cysts in corneal biopsy or scrapings. Medical treatment with topical propamidine, neomycin and imidazole antifungal agents may be successful, but corneal grafting is frequently necessary with a high risk of recurrent keratitis in the donor cornea.

Interstitial keratitis (Fig. 3.3.4)

Interstitial keratitis is a stromal vascularization and opacification and is usually associated with a systemic disease. Now uncommon, it is most often seen with congenital and acquired syphilis, other granulomatous diseases such as tuberculosis, herpes infections and onchocerciasis.

The initial findings are a kerato-uveitis followed by marked corneal vascularization. Late disease is characterized by ghost vessels and corneal opacification. Other stigmata of syphilis may be present, such as saddle nose, deafness, palatal perforation, and dental abnormalities. Syphilis serology should always be sought; the fluorescent treponemal antibody absorption test (FTA-ABS) is most likely to be positive in the presence of syphilitic interstitial keratitis.

Cogan's syndrome is painful interstitial keratitis and deafness with negative FTA-ABS. Nodular stromal keratitis is frequent and is often resistant to steroid therapy. The disease is thought to represent a vasculitis similar to polyarteritis nodosa.

Active interstitial keratitis should be treated with topical steroid and mydritatics, and appropriate systemic therapy. The chronic stromal scarring in late disease often necessitates penetrating keratoplasty.

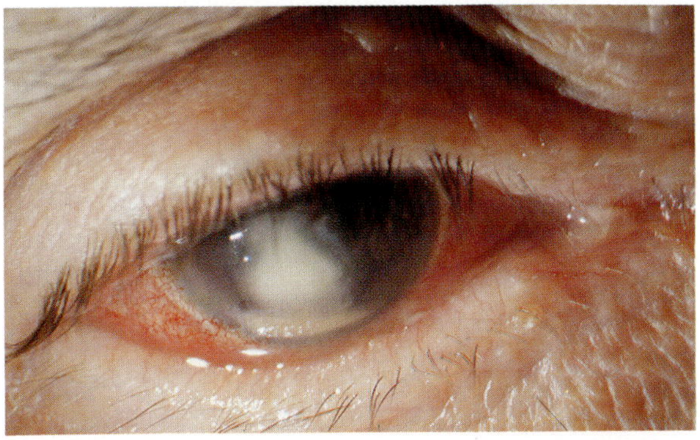

Fig. 3.3.1 Bacterial keratitis with associated hypopyon.

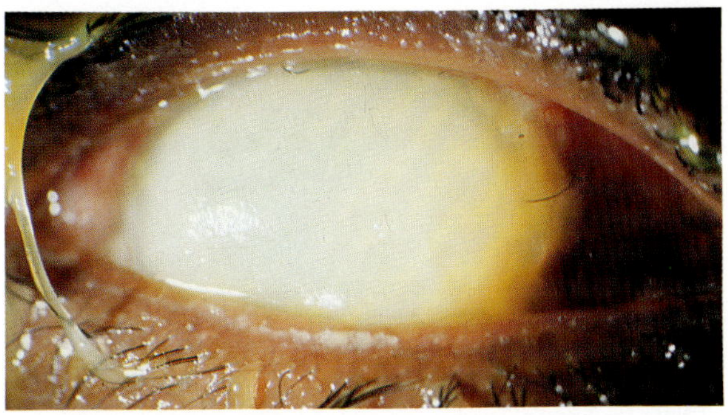

Fig. 3.3.2 Fungal keratitis (*Fusarium* spp.).

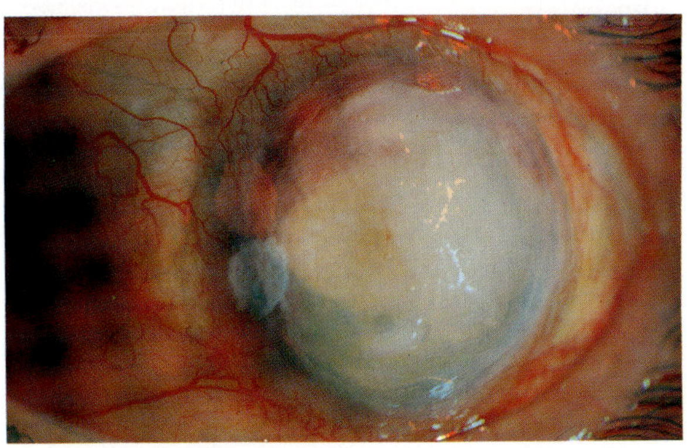

Fig. 3.3.3 Acanthamoeba keratitis.

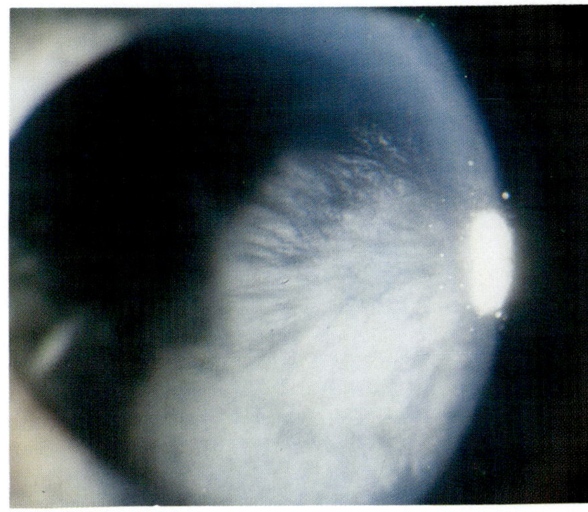

Fig. 3.3.4 Interstitial keratitis.

NON-INFECTIVE KERATITIS

The term 'non-infective keratitis' includes a variety of clinical appearances, some of which are characteristic of a specific disease whilst others are common to diverse pathologies. Accurate diagnosis is essential, not only to define management, but also to identify serious systemic disease whose first manifestation may be ocular.

A full medical as well as ocular history should therefore be taken, and examination should include attention to the ocular adnexae. Systemic examination directed in particular to abnormalities of the dermatologic, rheumatologic, respiratory and genito-urinary systems should be supported by relevant laboratory investigation.

The distinction between infective and non-infective keratitis is not always apparent, since infection may be present even when superficial corneal scraping demonstrates negative cultures. Corneal biopsy is a useful aid both in this situation and in the resolution of other diagnostic dilemmas.

Neurotrophic keratitis (Fig. 3.4.1)

Disturbance of normal corneal innervation by the ophthalmic branch of the trigeminal nerve is most frequently caused by infection with herpes zoster or simplex, but surgical transection of the nerve, compressive lesions, diabetes and — rarely — congenital abnormality, can also be responsible. The reduction in blink reflex leads to drying of the cornea, but in addition, the lack of a normal trophic influence of neurones on the cornea impairs normal epithelial function.

In neurotrophic keratitis, epithelial cell loss is followed by the development of indolent ulceration which may be refractory to treatment. Typically, the edges of the ulcer stain with Rose Bengal. Corneal sensation is reduced or absent.

Treatment should include topical lubricants together with partial tarsorrhaphy in severe cases. The use of collagenase inhibitors such as acetylcysteine is sometimes of benefit.

Exposure keratitis (Fig. 3.4.2)

This occurs in any condition leading to inadequate lid closure and consequent desiccation of the cornea. Dysthyroid eye disease and facial nerve paresis are the most frequent causes. Corneal changes are usually situated in the inferior third and include punctate erosions or, in more extreme cases, ulceration and thinning. Secondary bacterial infection is not uncommon.

Treatment should be directed at the cause of the exposure and may include tarsorrhaphy for facial palsy, or repositioning of retracted eyelids in dysthyroid eye disease. In addition, topical lubricants should be liberally applied, and any infection treated. If development of exposure can be anticipated (for example, at the time of neurosurgical resection of an acoustic neuroma involving the seventh nerve), then a prophylactic tarsorrhaphy is indicated.

Superior limbic keratoconjunctivitis (Fig. 3.4.3)

This is a condition affecting the cornea adjacent to the superior limbus, with inflammation of the adjacent bulbar conjunctiva and apposing tarsal conjunctiva. It is seen in association with hyperthyroidism and hyperparathyroidism, as well as keratoconjunctivitis sicca.

The corneal change is usually that of fine punctate epitheliopathy, often associated with filamentary keratitis. Although the pathogenesis of the condition remains speculative, it is most likely a mechanical effect caused by the abnormal movement of the upper eyelid in tight apposition to the superior bulbar conjunctiva.

Treatment should include application of topical lubricants, topical vitamin A or *N*-acetylcysteine, but if this is not successful resection of the superior bulbar conjunctiva or its treatment with silver nitrate may help. Bandage contact lenses provide temporary relief.

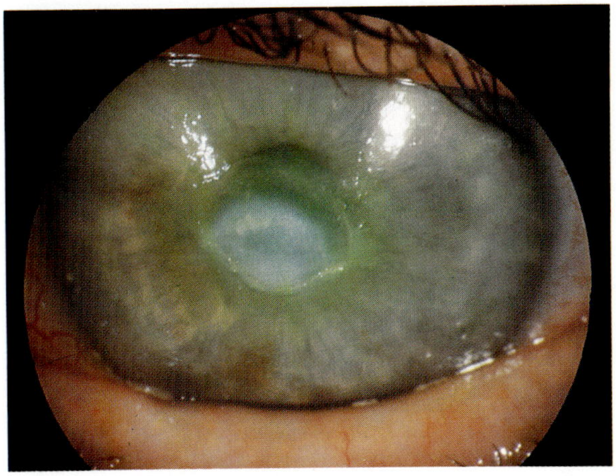

Fig. 3.4.1 Neurotrophic keratitis.

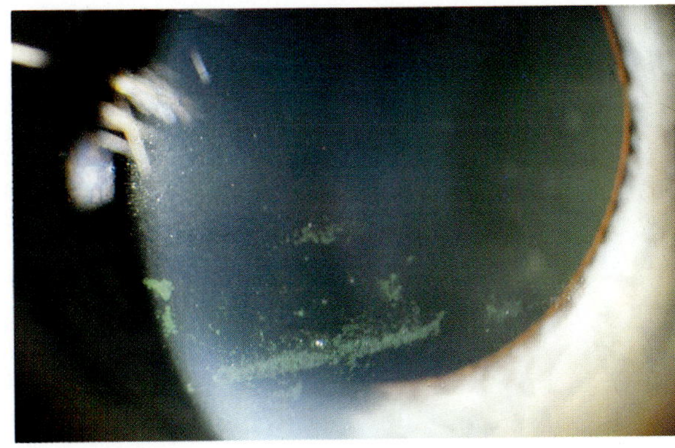

Fig. 3.4.2 Exposure keratitis.

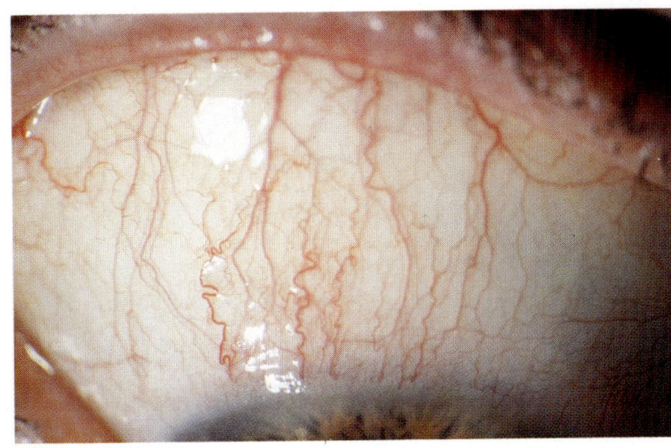

Fig. 3.4.3 Superior limbic keratoconjunctivitis.

Marginal keratis (catarrhal ulcer) (Fig. 3.4.4)

This is a hypersensitivity reaction to bacterial exotoxin, usually associated with chronic staphylococcal lid disease. It is characterized by a small subepithelial infiltrate which develops in the peripheral cornea, but separated from the limbus by a 2 mm clear zone. Breakdown of the overlying epithelium occurs several days later, and an adjacent limbal inflammation is typical.

Differentiation of the condition from peripheral herpes simplex keratitis, which begins with epithelial breakdown and is followed by infiltrate, is important since marginal keratitis responds well to topical steroid, which is contraindicated in herpes simplex infection. Treatment of the blepharitis is an important component of the management of marginal keratitis.

Mooren's ulcer (Fig. 3.4.5)

This is a destructive condition of the peripheral cornea, characterized by severe pain and progressive corneal melting. Two forms exist, one affecting those in their fifth decade, or beyond; this is unilateral and usually responds well to treatment. The other affects younger individuals and is often bilateral, relentless and unresponsive to treatment.

The condition begins as a peripheral stromal infiltrate which is followed by overlying epithelial loss contiguous with the limbus. The ulcer spreads centrally and circumferentially, and is characterized by an overhanging edge on its corneal side. Thinning and vascularization may progress to perforation (Fig. 3.4.6).

Initial treatment should include topical cycloplegics and intensive topical steroids. Application of a bandage contact lens may relieve discomfort and prevent perforation. Conjunctival resection, which removes local collagenases, immunoglobulins and complement which mediate the keratolysis, is successful in some cases. Patients unresponsive to these measures require treatment with systemic steroids and immunosuppressives; these include cyclophosphamide, methotrexate, azathioprine and cyclosporin A.

Tectonic keratoplasty or epikeratoplasty are necessary in cases of extreme thinning with threatened or actual perforation, but recurrence of the disease in the graft is common.

Rheumatoid arthritis

This disease produces widespread immune-complex-mediated inflammation, and has a number of ocular manifestations. The typical systemic features are morning stiffness, joint pain with characteristic deformities and subcutaneous rheumatoid nodules found predominantly at pressure points such as the elbows and ischial tuberosities. There may be pulmonary or cardiovascular involvement.

Keratoconjunctivitis sicca is seen in association with rheumatoid arthritis and is discussed in Section 2.

Peripheral corneal thinning (contact lens cornea) (Fig. 3.4.7)

This is seen in longstanding rheumatoid disease and appears as a ring of thinned peripheral cornea, without any adjacent limbal inflammation. The remaining cornea is of normal thickness and, though the condition is normally not aggressive in behaviour, it can progress to corneal melting.

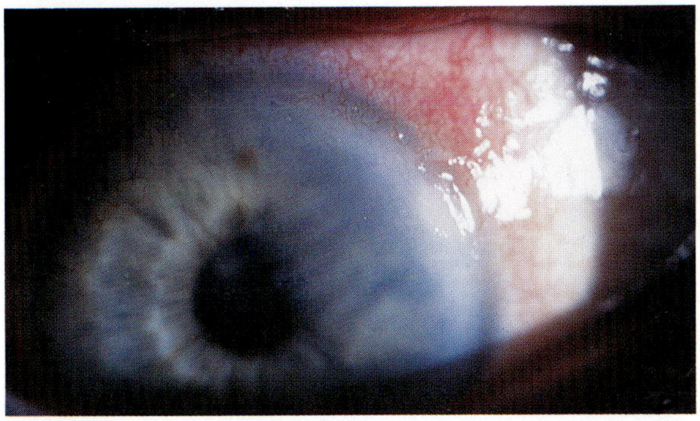

Fig. 3.4.4 Marginal keratitis.

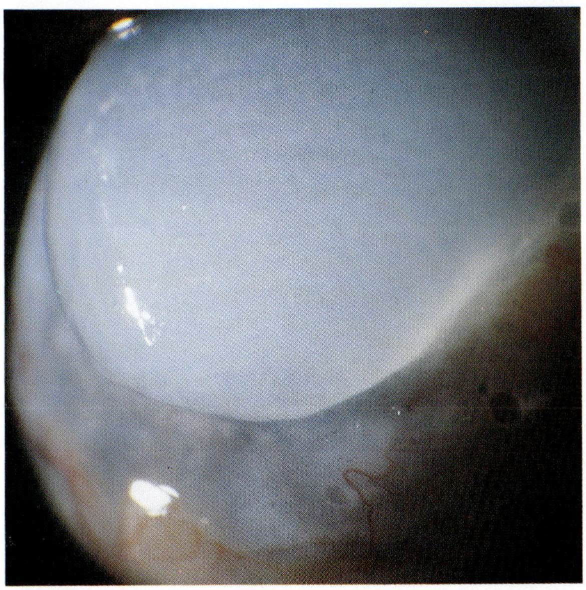

Fig. 3.4.5 Mooren's ulcer.

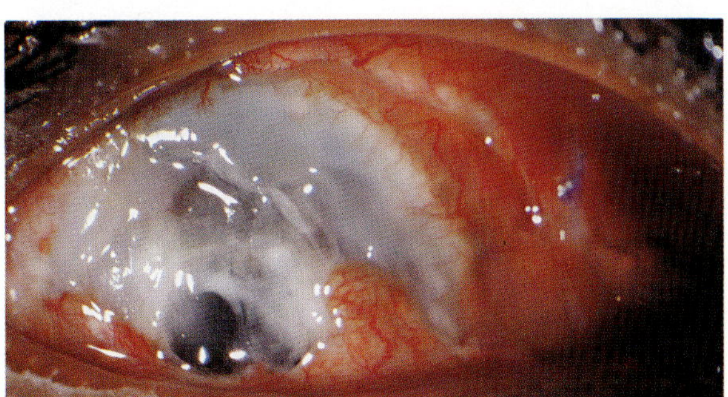

Fig. 3.4.6 Corneal perforation secondary to Mooren's ulcer.

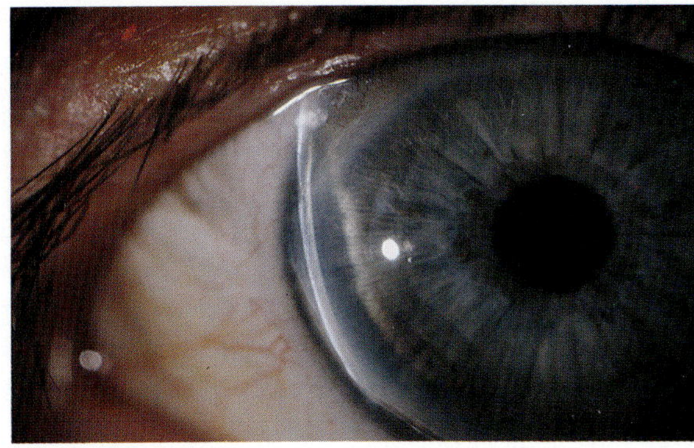

Fig. 3.4.7 Peripheral corneal thinning.

Peripheral corneal melting (Fig. 3.4.8)

This is usually associated with limbal inflammatory activity, with or without scleritis, and is due to deposition of immune complexes in the limbal vasculature which causes a vasculitis with leakage of inflammatory substances. In addition, immune complex deposition in the cornea leads to melting through activation of the classic complement pathway. Other vasculitides, such as Wegener's granulomatosis, polyarteritis nodosa and systemic lupus erythematosus can produce similar peripheral ulceration and it is important to identify these conditions, which may be life-threatening. The skin should be examined for features such as erythema nodosum (Fig. 3.4.9) or microinfarcts which may reflect systemic vasculitis. In addition, full blood count and erythrocyte sedimentation rate, rheumatoid factor and circulating immune complex assay, chest and sinus X-ray and urinalysis should be undertaken. Systemic vasculitic processes require immunosuppressive therapy, following which there is often an improvement in the corneal condition.

Topical therapy should include the treatment of any associated dry eye state or secondary infection, but steroids should be avoided. Conjunctival resection is of benefit in some cases, and tectonic grafting may be necessary.

Rosacea keratitis (Fig. 3.4.10)

The cornea is frequently involved in rosacea secondary to the lid disease. A characteristic peripheral corneal infiltration, vascularization and thinning is seen. Active keratitis responds well to topical steroids, but these patients are particularly prone to rapid corneal thinning and spontaneous corneal perforation may occur (Fig. 3.4.11). Tectonic grafting or surgery for astigmatism may be required.

Ectodermal dysplasia (Fig. 3.4.12)

This is a widespread maldevelopment of ectodermal structures, which can occur in two forms: the hypohidrotic condition, associated with sweat gland hypoplasia, and the hidrotic form in which there is normal gland function.

Common to both are the dental anomalies of hypodontia or anodontia, hyperkeratosis of the skin of the palms and soles, hair loss and an abnormal facies.

Corneal changes develop both secondary to gland hypoplasia, and as part of the primary ectodermal abnormality. They include punctate epithelial keratitis, drying of the cornea, secondary infection, epithelial cysts, and widespread bilateral pannus. Cataract is also associated.

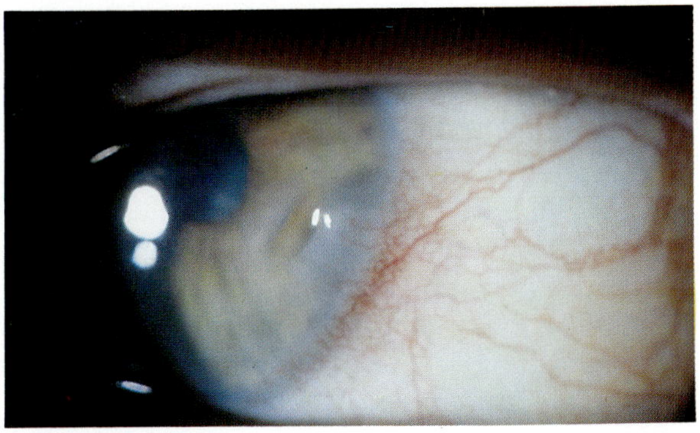

Fig. 3.4.8 Peripheral corneal melting.

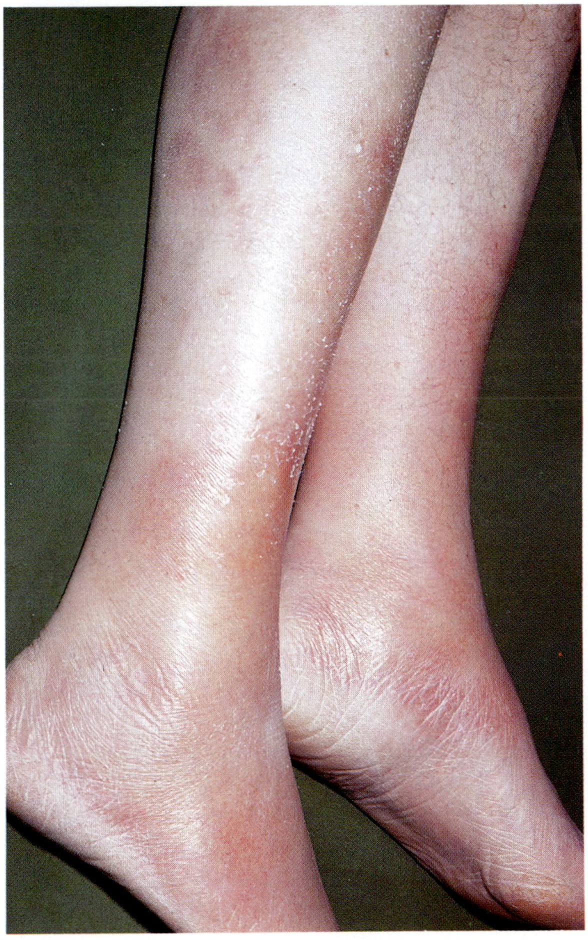

Fig. 3.4.9 Erythema nodosum of both legs.

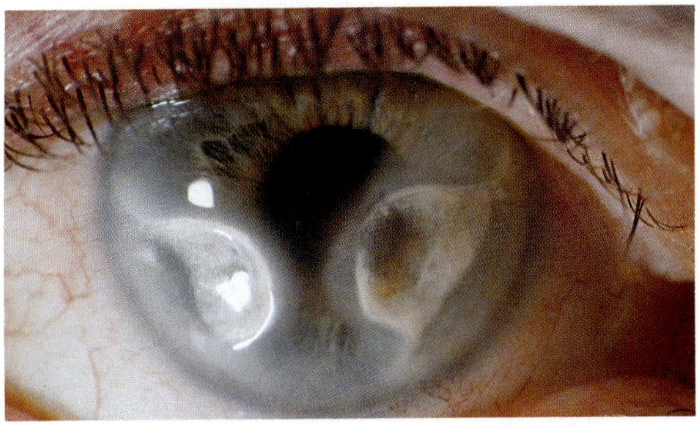

Fig. 3.4.10 Rosacea keratitis.

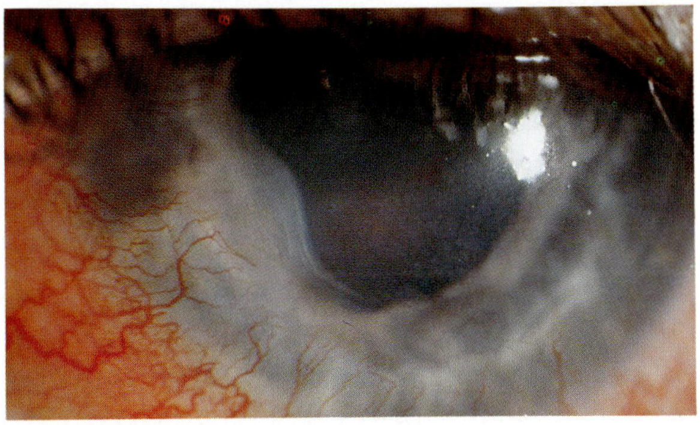

Fig. 3.4.11 Corneal melting and perforation secondary to rosacea keratitis.

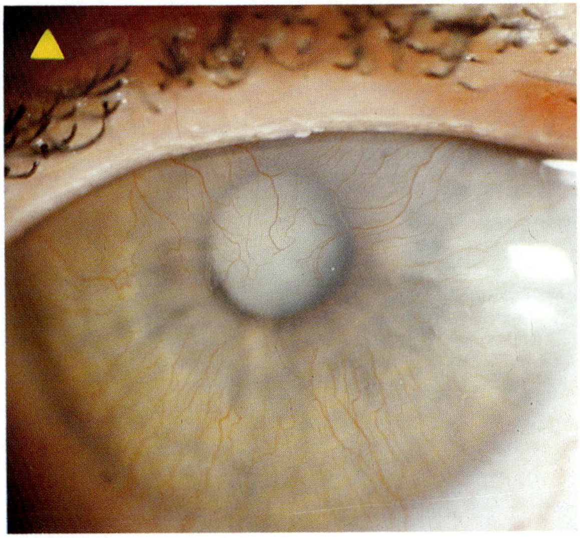

Fig. 3.4.12 Extensive corneal pannus in ectodermal dysplasia.

CORNEAL DYSTROPHIES

Corneal dystrophies are inherited, bilateral and isolated ocular abnormalities. The mode of inheritance is autosomal dominant in all except macular dystrophy. They are conveniently grouped anatomically according to the site of the primary defect, although a number of corneal layers may be involved.

The associated symptoms are variable; many patients are symptom free, whilst others experience pain from recurrent epithelial loss and reduced vision due to corneal opacification. Corneal grafting may be necessary but recurrence of the original pathology can occur in the graft.

Epithelial dystrophy

Meesman's dystrophy (Fig. 3.5.1)

This is a rare and frequently asymptomatic dystrophy characterized by multiple intraepithelial cysts containing inclusion material the nature of which is undetermined. Recurrent erosion can develop late in the disease, but treatment is rarely required.

Reis–Bücklers' dystrophy (Fig. 3.5.2)

This usually presents with pain and photophobia in childhood, due to recurrent epithelial loss, which is followed by scarring in Bowman's membrane. Eventually the erosive episodes subside and vision is reduced because of corneal scarring and resultant astigmatism. At this stage corneal grafting may be necessary.

Map-dot-fingerprint dystrophy (Cogan's dystrophy)

This is the commonest of the epithelial dystrophies. Recurrent epithelial erosions develop, most probably secondary to an abnormality of the basement membrane (Fig. 3.5.3). These usually occur first in the fourth decade of life.

The dystrophy can adopt a variety of appearances, which change as opacities come and go spontaneously. The three typical forms adopted give their names to the dystrophy: map lesions, which are diffuse grey areas; dot lesions, which are scattered intraepithelial cysts (Fig. 3.5.4); fingerprint lesions (Fig. 3.5.5). The dot lesions can also be found in the dystrophic post-traumatic recurrent abrasion syndrome.

Management is aimed at relief of the acute episodes and establishment of epithelial integrity. Hyperosmotic agents, topical lubricants and contact lenses may reduce the frequency of epithelial loss. Superficial keratectomy can be successful in establishing a normal epithelial basement membrane and epithelial stability.

Stromal dystrophy

Granular dystrophy (Fig. 3.5.6)

Symptoms appear late in this stromal dystrophy, in which fine discrete white dots and lines occur in the anterior central stroma. These progress to breadcrumb-like opacities, but do not extend to the periphery. Visual loss is usually mild until late in the disease, and epithelial erosion is unusual.

The proteinaceous material deposited in the stroma stains red with Masson trichrome (Fig. 3.5.7).

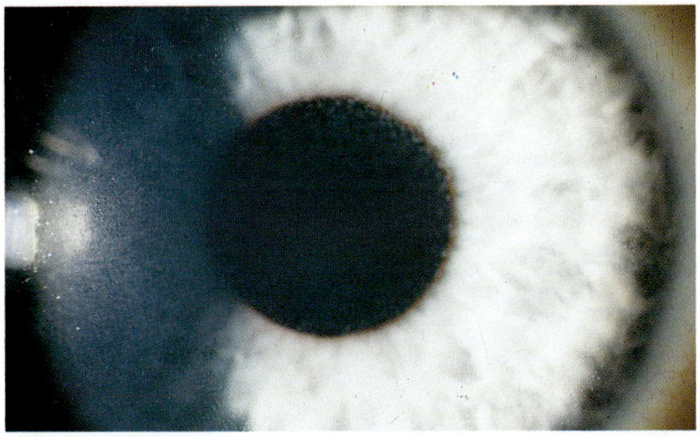

Fig. 3.5.1 Meesman's dystrophy.

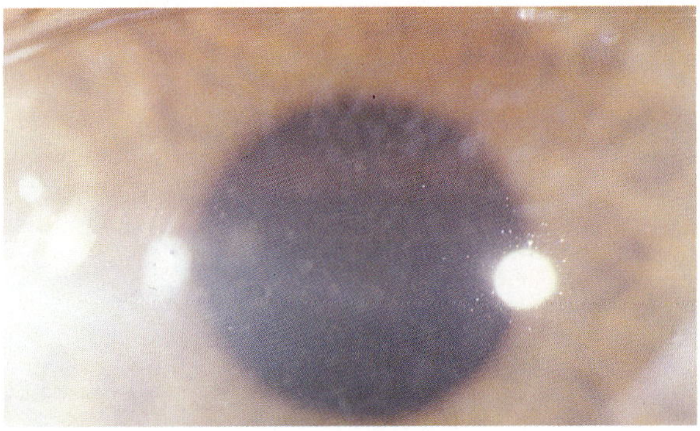

Fig. 3.5.2 Reis–Bücklers' dystrophy.

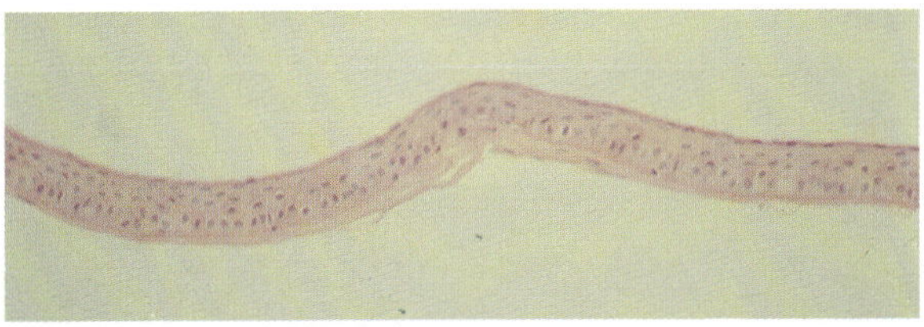

Fig. 3.5.3 Corneal epithelium stained with haematoxylin and eosin with abnormal basement membrane in map–dot–fingerprint dystrophy.

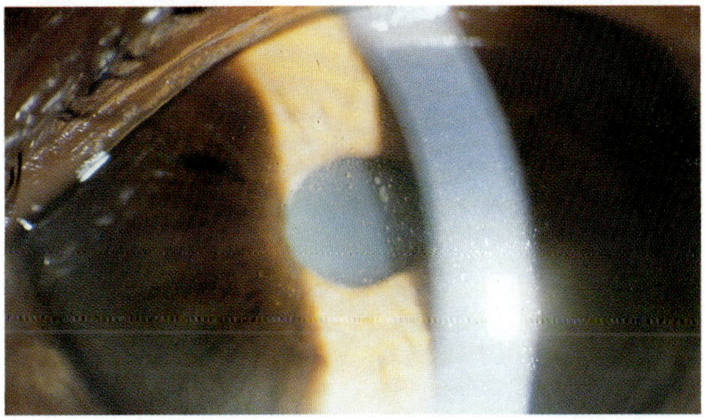

Fig. 3.5.4 Map–dot–fingerprint dystrophy: dot lesions.

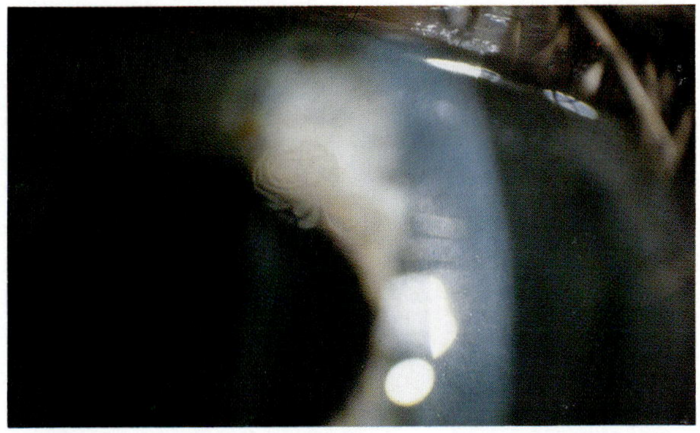

Fig. 3.5.5 Map–dot–fingerprint dystrophy: fingerprint lesion.

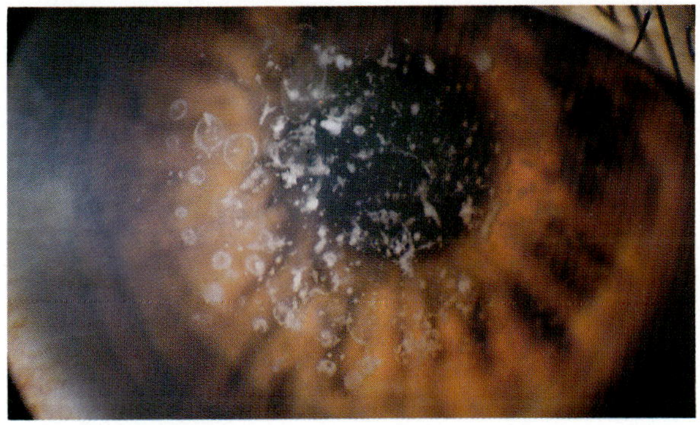

Fig. 3.5.6 Granular dystrophy.

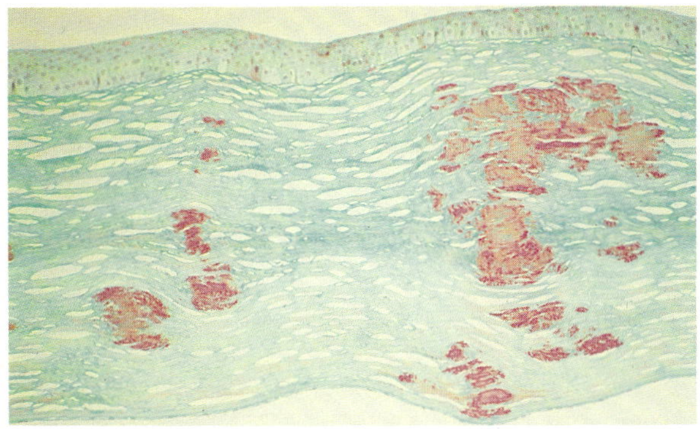

Fig. 3.5.7 Section of cornea with granular dystrophy stained with Masson trichrome.

Macular dystrophy (Fig. 3.5.8)

This is inherited in an autosomal recessive manner. The initial feature is of a stromal haze which is followed by the development of ill-defined stromal nodules that extend forwards into the epithelium. Epithelial loss is frequent and vision is lost due to corneal opacification. The lesions characteristically extend out to the corneal periphery.

Corneal grafting is usually required, and the disease frequently recurs in the graft. Histological staining of the cornea demonstrates the presence of glycosaminoglycan (Fig. 3.5.9).

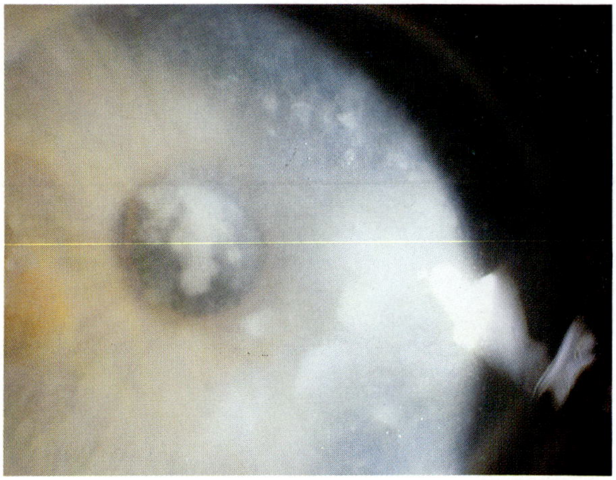

Fig. 3.5.8 Macular dystrophy.

Lattice dystrophy (Fig. 3.5.10)

Epithelial loss is frequent in this dystrophy, where typically filamentous branching lines are found in the central corneal stroma due to amyloid deposition. These deposits appear orange-red with Congo Red stain (Fig. 3.5.11), and they exhibit birefringence with polarized light.

Systemic amyloidosis can occasionally show mild lattice lines within the cornea.

Fig. 3.5.9 Macular dystrophy with abnormal deposits in stroma stained with Alcian Blue.

Schnyder's central crystalline dystrophy (Fig. 3.5.12)

This is characterized by crystalline deposits of cholesterol and neutral fats in the stroma (Fig. 3.5.13). Some patients have an associated hyperlipidaemia. Corneal grafting may be necessary if the visual axis is involved.

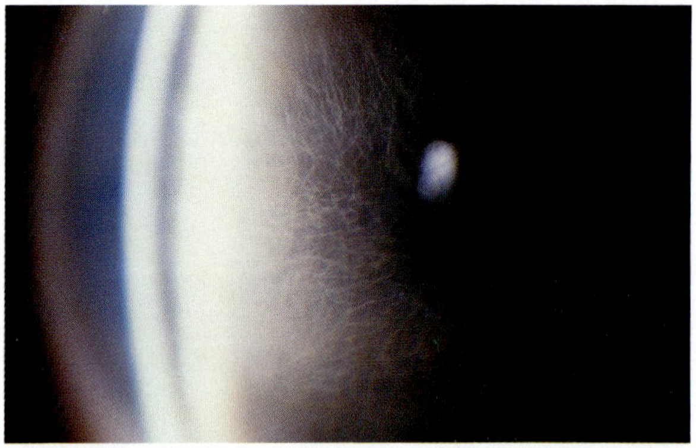

Fig. 3.5.10 Lattice dystrophy.

Endothelial dystrophy

Fuchs' endothelial dystrophy

This is common, and frequently symptomatic. Three stages of the disease are recognized: cornea guttata, corneal oedema and corneal scarring.

Cornea guttata (Fig. 3.5.14) produces no symptoms. It is recognized as a stippling, which is often pigmented, of the posterior corneal surface. Dark holes may also be seen. Specular microscopy highlights the severity of the endothelial disorder. Descemet's membrane becomes thickened and has multiple warty excrescences that project towards the anterior chamber (Fig. 3.5.15).

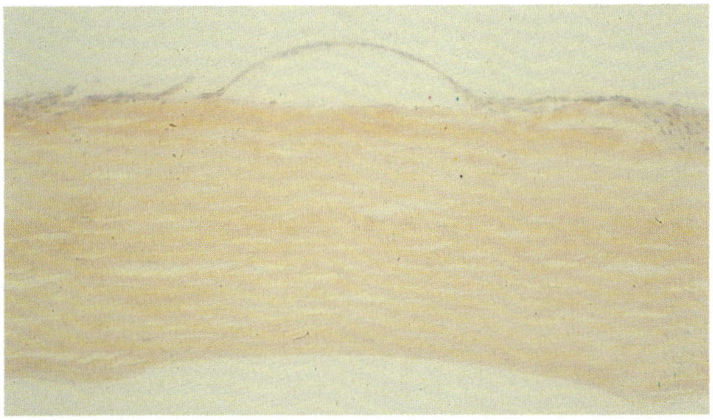

Fig. 3.5.11 Lattice dystrophy with abnormal deposits stained with Congo Red.

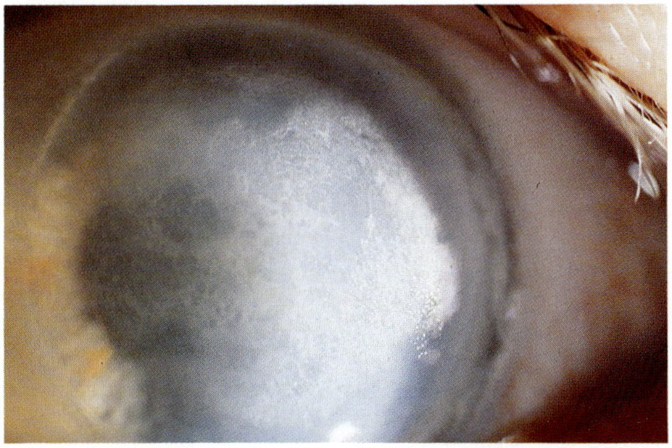

Fig. 3.5.12 Schnyder's central crystalline dystrophy.

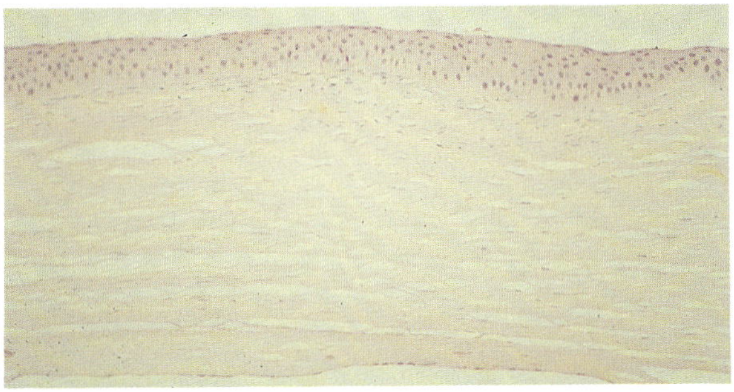

Fig. 3.5.13 Schnyder's central crystalline dystrophy stained with haematoxylin and eosin. Abnormal clefts in stroma that contained lipid.

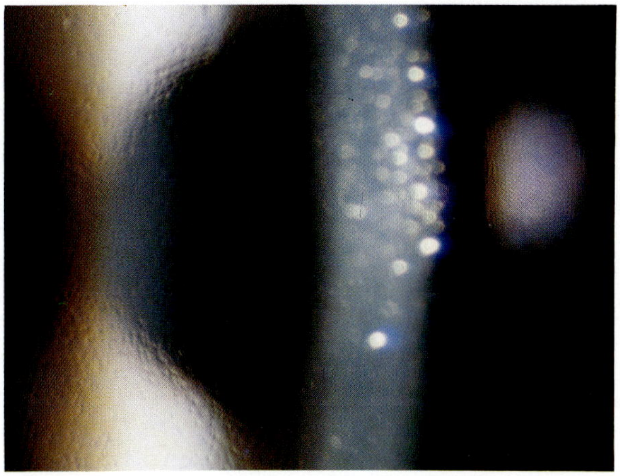

Fig. 3.5.14 Cornea guttata demonstrated by retro-illumination.

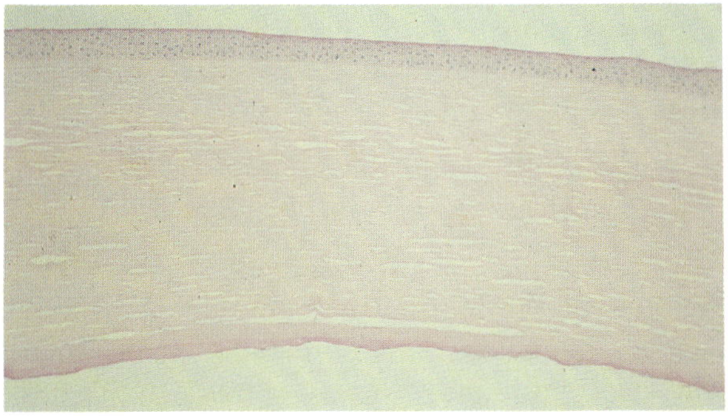

Fig. 3.5.15 Fuchs' endothelial dystrophy. Cornea stained with periodic acid–Schiff showing absence of endothelial cells and thickened Descemet's membrane.

Corneal oedema (Fig. 3.5.16) involves initially the stroma, and tends to present first following prolonged eye closure when corneal oxygenation and tear film evaporation are reduced. Corneal thickness increases, and folds develop in Descemet's membrane. Epithelial oedema leads to painful erosions, and the development of bullae.

Scarring and vascularization allow some relief of pain and discomfort, but vision remains poor (Fig. 3.5.17). Dystrophic calcification late in the disease is common.

Early Fuchs' dystrophy requires no treatment, but caution must be exercised in considering such patients for cataract surgery, which may precipitate corneal decompensation (Fig. 3.5.18). Early stromal oedema may be helped by hyperosmotic agents and the use of warm dry air to aid evaporation. Advanced disease requires corneal grafting.

Posterior polymorphous dystrophy (Fig. 3.5.19)

This dystrophy is also associated with abnormalities of the iris and anterior chamber angle. It is frequently asymptomatic. Endothelial vacuoles and polymorphic figures are seen, together with peripheral anterior synechiae, irido-corneal adhesions, and ectropion uveae. Histologically the endothelium assumes the appearances of epithelial cells (Fig. 3.5.20). Treatment is unnecessary unless glaucoma or corneal oedema develop.

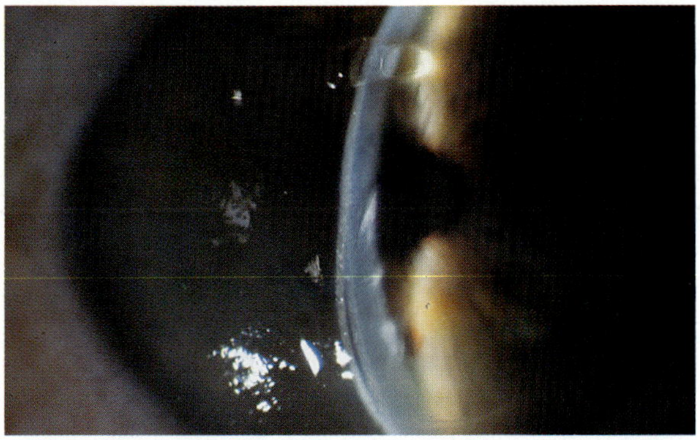

Fig. 3.5.16 Corneal oedema with bullae, secondary to Fuchs' dystrophy. Note folds in Descemet's membrane.

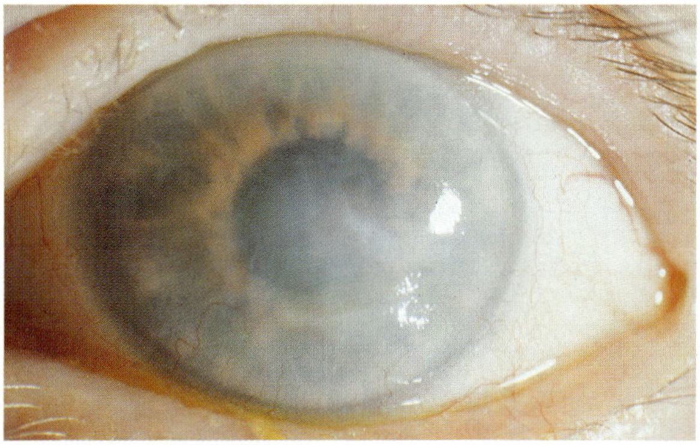

Fig. 3.5.17 Scarring of the cornea in Fuchs' dystrophy.

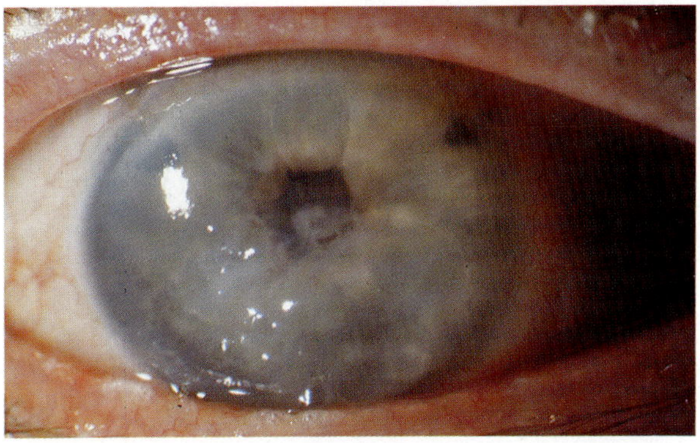

Fig. 3.5.18 Corneal decompensation following cataract surgery in Fuchs' dystrophy.

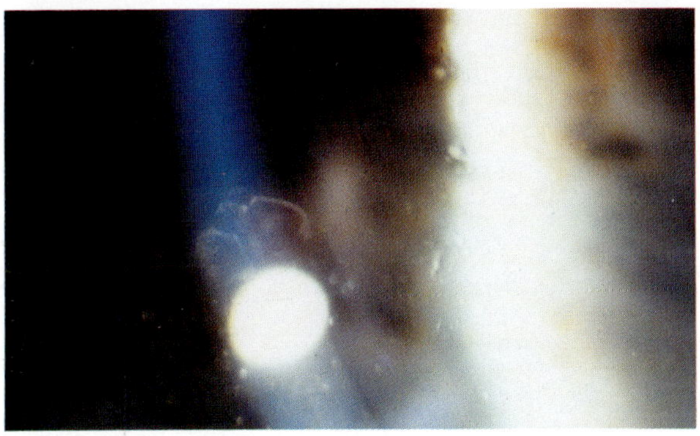

Fig. 3.5.19 Posterior polymorphous dystrophy.

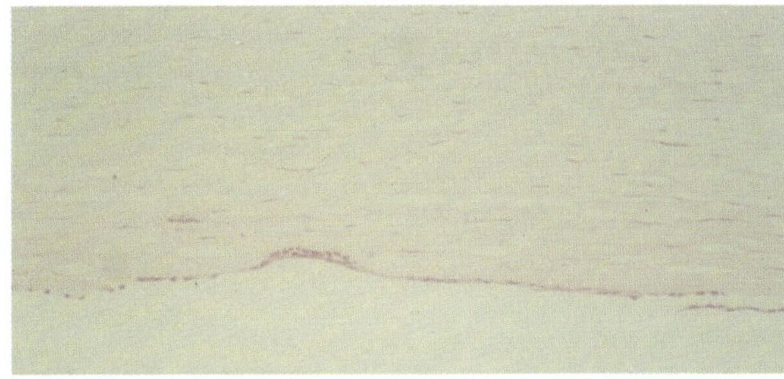

Fig. 3.5.20 Posterior polymorphous dystrophy. Cornea stained with haematoxylin and eosin showing epithelial character of endothelial cells.

ECTATIC CORNEAL DYSTROPHIES

Keratoconus (Fig. 3.6.1)

Keratoconus is a non-inflammatory disorder of the cornea which leads to bilateral, asymmetrical ectasia and mainly central thinning. Although it may be congenital, the normal onset of symptoms is around puberty. The cornea assumes a conical shape, the initial presenting feature often being irregular astigmatism and myopia.

The fundamental pathology of the condition remains undetermined. It has variously been regarded as a neurocristopathy or a biochemical abnormality of stromal collagen. A number of ocular and systemic associations exist.

Fleischer ring (Fig. 3.6.2)

This is a deposition of iron seen at the base of the corneal protrusion in keratoconus. Haemosiderin is deposited within and between the epithelial cells in a (usually incomplete) ring.

Vogt's striae (Fig. 3.6.3)

These are vertical striae which develop in the deep stroma and Descemet's membrane, and are an early sign of keratoconus.

Stromal scarring (Fig. 3.6.4)

This may develop in the anterior stroma following rupture of Bowman's membrane, and its repair with scar tissue, or deeper in the stroma, secondary to Descemet's membrane rupture. Scarring may flatten the cornea, and so even improve acuity, but if the visual axis is involved, vision is severely compromised.

Corneal hydrops (Fig. 3.6.5)

This is an acute corneal oedema resulting from tearing of Descemet's membrane. The oedema usually clears spontaneously as endothelial cells bridge the tear and deposit a new membrane. However, if the tear is close to the visual axis, the ensuing scarring necessitates penetrating keratoplasty. This should be deferred until the oedema has settled, which usually occurs within 3 to 4 months. Perforation is exceedingly rare. Hydrops occurs more frequently in keratoconus associated with Down's syndrome.

Munson's sign (Fig. 3.6.6)

Extreme distortion of the cornea leads to distortion of the lower lid margin profile on downgaze. This phenomenon is termed Munson's sign.

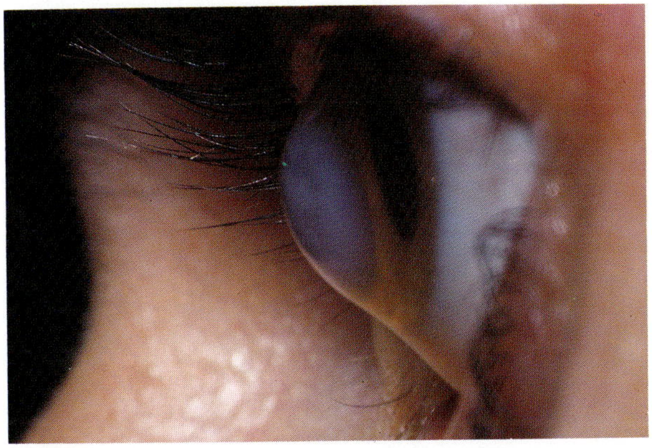

Fig. 3.6.1 Keratoconus showing central corneal decompensation.

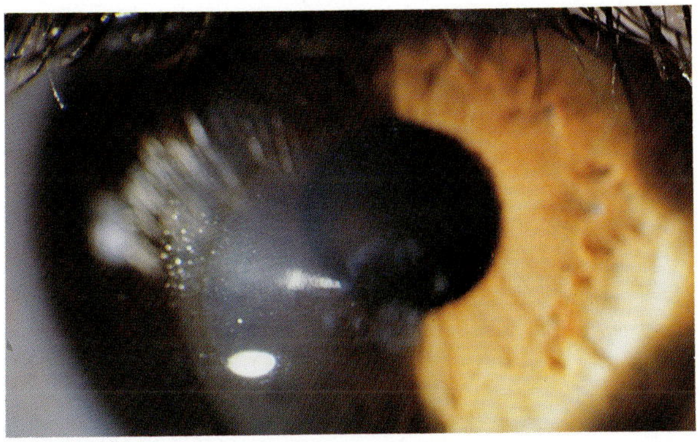

Fig. 3.6.2 Fleischer ring at base of cone in keratoconus.

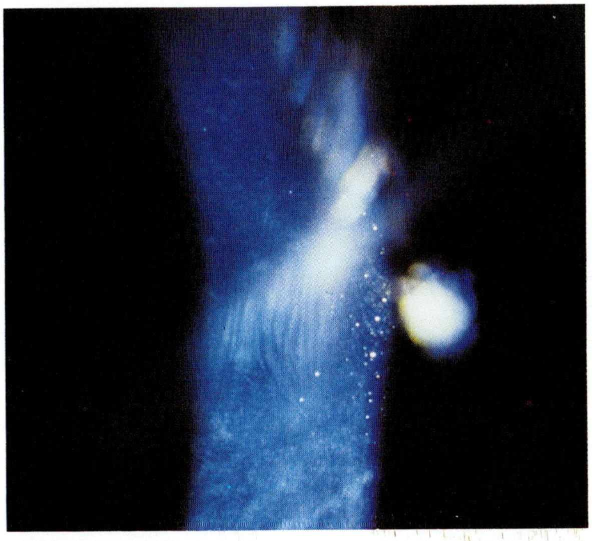

Fig. 3.6.3 Vogt's striae.

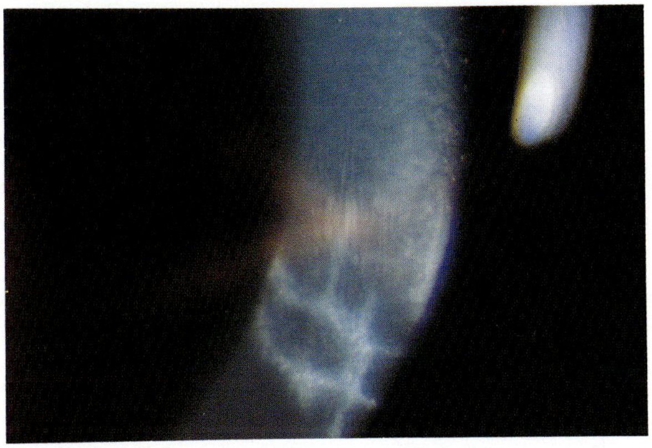

Fig. 3.6.4 Stromal scarring in keratoconus.

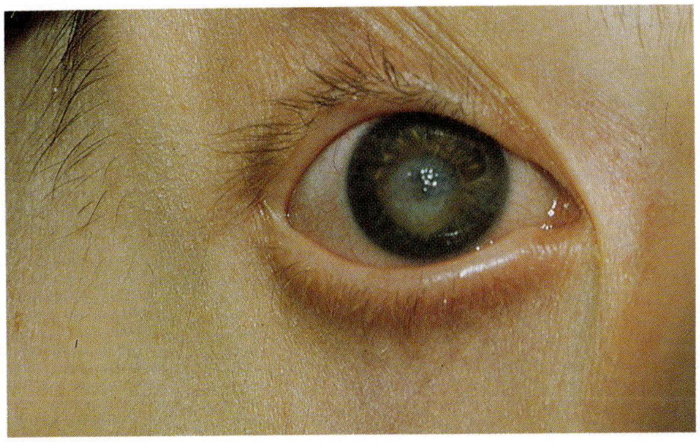

Fig. 3.6.5 Acute corneal hydrops.

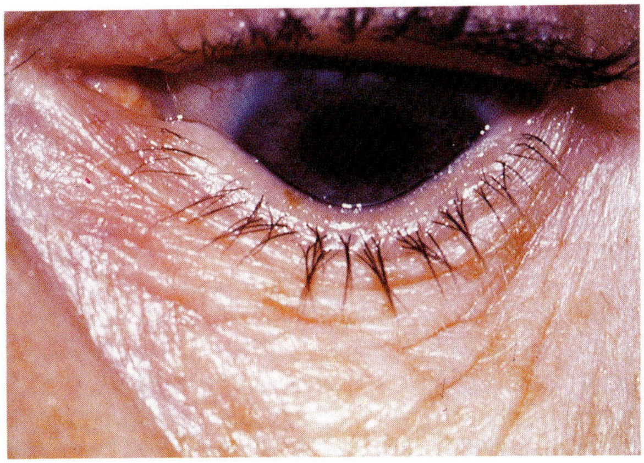

Fig. 3.6.6 Munson's sign.

Histology (Fig. 3.6.7)

Histological sections of corneas with keratoconus show marked variation in thickness, often with thinned areas adjacent to areas of marked oedema. Breaks in Descemet's membrane are often filled with collagenous material and PAS positive granular deposits are seen. Downgrowths of epithelium into Bowman's membrane may be seen, as well as breaks in Descemet's membrane.

Associations

Keratoconus is associated particularly with atopic disease (Fig. 3.6.8) such as asthma, eczema and hayfever, as well as Down's syndrome and a number of connective tissue disorders. These include Ehlers–Danlos syndrome and mitral valve prolapse, and reflect a collagen abnormality common to both the cornea and other tissues.

Associations exist also with a number of ocular diseases, such as Leber's congenital amaurosis, retinitis pigmentosa, posterior polymorphous dystrophy and endothelial dystrophy.

Treatment

Early keratoconus can be treated with spectacles alone, but the disease soon requires contact lens correction to achieve good acuity. Because of the high astigmatism, it is usually necessary to use a rigid lens, and gas-permeable lenses are well suited. Techniques such as the 'piggy-back' combination of a hard lens fitted over a large soft contact lens, or soft lenses with an integral hard centre, may be useful in more severe cases. Advanced disease requires surgical correction. This usually comprises penetrating keratoplasty (Fig. 3.6.9), although epikeratoplasty and lamellar keratoplasty can be used for keratoconus without extensive scarring.

Keratoglobus (Fig. 3.6.10)

This is a rare, bilateral, non-inflammatory disorder in which a diffuse thinning of the cornea leads to its assuming a globular shape.

The stroma tends to remain clear, although acute hydrops can occur. Spontaneous perforation is not infrequent and is difficult to treat owing to the extreme thinning. The disease is sometimes seen in relatives of patients with keratoconus, although no hereditary pattern has been clearly identified.

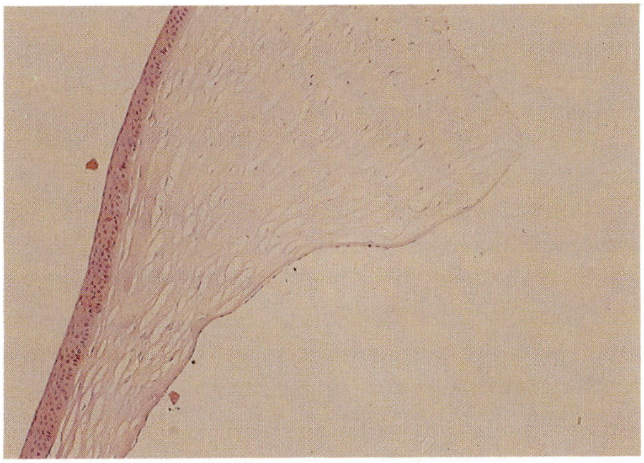

Fig. 3.6.7 Histological section of cornea with keratoconus (stained with haematoxylin and eosin).

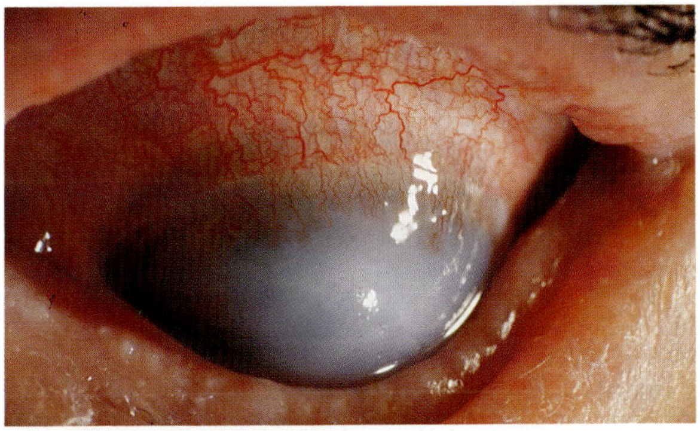

Fig. 3.6.8 Keratoconus associated with eczematous lid disease.

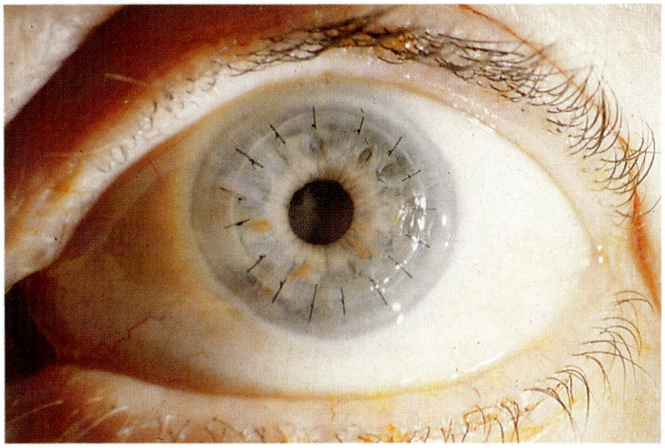

Fig. 3.6.9 Penetrating keratoplasty for keratoconus.

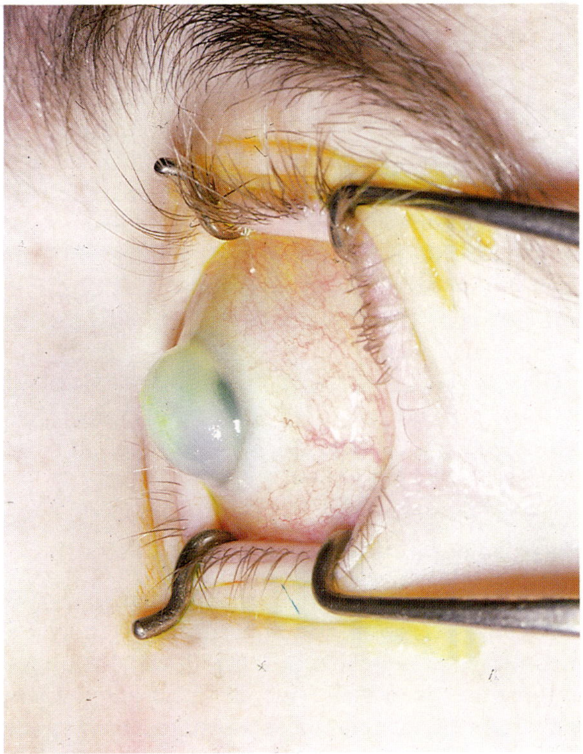

Fig. 3.6.10 Keratoglobus.

CORNEAL DEGENERATIONS

Limbal girdle of Vogt (Fig. 3.7.1)

This is a crescent-shaped degenerative change situated in the interpalpebral zone, parallel to, and continuous with, the limbus. It reflects subepithelial hyaline degeneration similar to that seen in pingueculae and pterygia. Visual acuity is not affected, and it should be regarded as an involutional change.

The typical limbal girdle of Vogt as described is often termed 'type II'. The type I girdle, in which there is a lucid zone between it and the limbus, is less common.

Band keratopathy (Fig. 3.7.2)

This is a deposition of the hydroxyapatite crystal of calcium carbonate in the cornea. It may be secondary to pre-existing local disease, such as chronic uveitis or glaucoma, or to raised circulating levels of calcium or phosphate, as seen in sarcoidosis, hyperparathyroidism, and metastatic disease.

The deposition occurs in the interpalpebral zone, and commences at the limbus to move centrally. A clear zone separates it from the limbus. Treatment is required only if the deposition encroaches upon the visual axis, and should be the application of 0.05 mol/l EDTA to the cornea after removal of the epithelium in the affected area, followed by scraping of the deposited calcium.

Salzmann's nodular degeneration (Fig. 3.7.3)

This can occur as a primary disease, or secondary to previous ocular inflammatory disorders such as phlyctenular keratitis, trachoma, measles or vernal keratitis.

A number of nodules of hypertrophic collagen are deposited beneath Bowman's membrane; this elevates the epithelium. A degree of localized corneal vascularization may be associated. Visual acuity is not normally significantly reduced, but if a nodule is situated axially, superficial keratectomy may be required. Very extensive or recurrent disease may necessitate lamellar or even penetrating keratoplasty.

Lipid keratopathy (Fig. 3.7.4)

This is a focal deposition of lipid in the corneal stroma, which normally is secondary to previous corneal vascularization. It is situated around the vessels and probably reflects their abnormal permeability. Repeated argon-laser treatment of the involved vessels will often lead to resorption of the lipid.

A primary form of the condition also exists in which a bilateral ring-shaped deposition is seen, similar in appearance to arcus senilis, but more extensive.

Corneal mosaic (Fig. 3.7.5)

A number of different corneal mosaic patterns have been described which are usually involutional in origin. Peripheral mosaic pattern is a symmetrical, age-related criss-cross appearance in Descemet's membrane and the overlying stroma. 'Crocodile shagreen' may occur either at the level of Bowman's membrane (anterior) or more deeply to involve Descemet's membrane and deep stroma (posterior). François dystrophy is a central corneal clouding affecting the deep stroma and is also regarded as a mosaic. Visual acuity is not affected. Mosaic patterns can also be produced by a reduction in corneal tension, as may occur in hypotony, through relaxation of Bowman's membrane.

Cornea farinata (Fig. 3.7.6)

This is a benign appearance of a fine, flour-like dusting of the posterior corneal stroma which is normally bilateral and does not affect visual acuity.

It probably reflects lipofuscin deposition, and as such, a mild degenerative change. The distribution is within the central portion of the cornea.

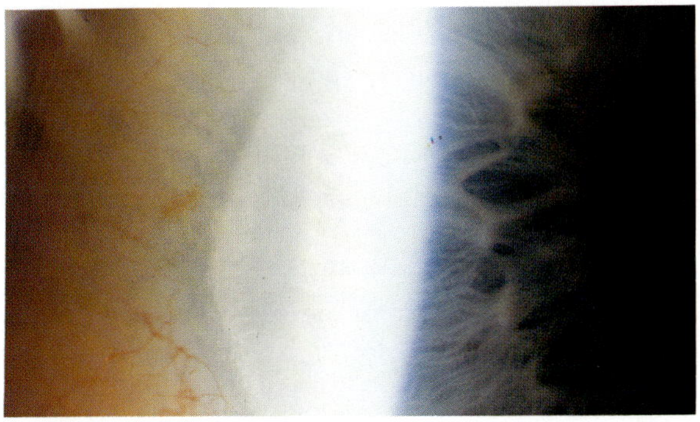

Fig. 3.7.1 Limbal girdle of Vogt.

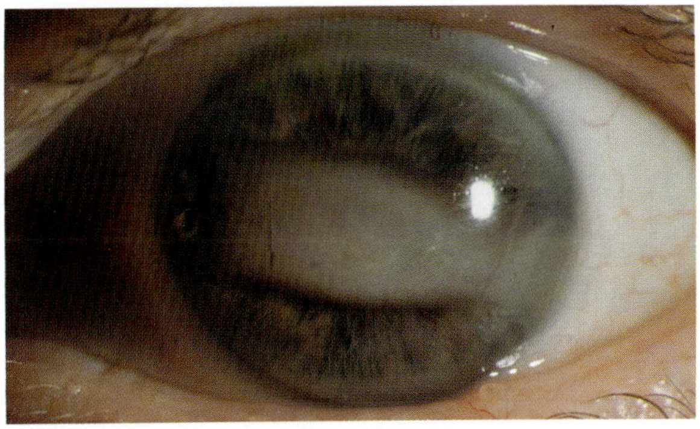

Fig. 3.7.2 Band keratopathy.

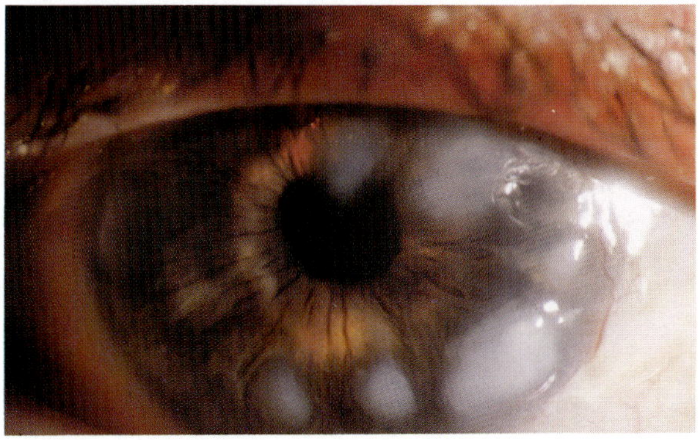

Fig. 3.7.3 Salzmann's nodular degeneration.

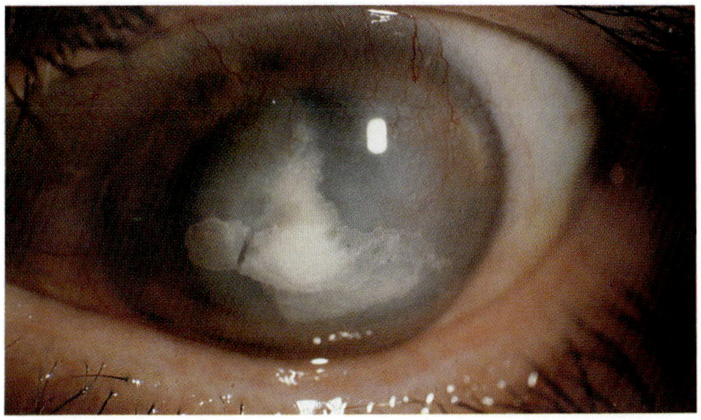

Fig. 3.7.4 Lipid keratopathy secondary to herpes simplex infection.

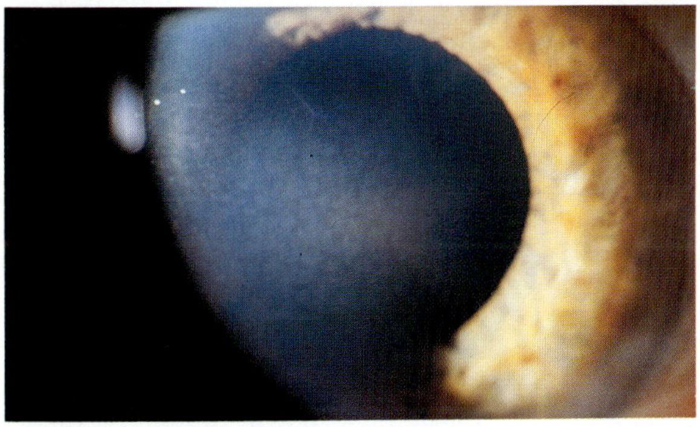

Fig. 3.7.5 Corneal mosaic.

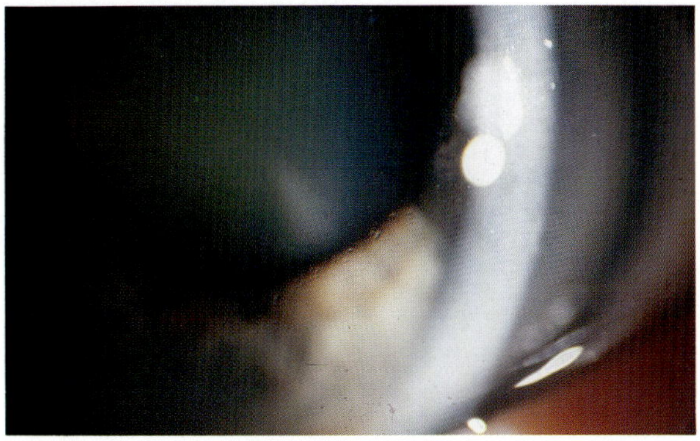

Fig. 3.7.6 Cornea farinata.

Terrien's marginal degeneration (Fig. 3.7.7)

This condition can occur at any age, and is usually bilateral though asymmetrical. Marginal thinning of the stroma, covered by an intact epithelium, occurs concentric with the limbus, separated from it by a narrow, uninvolved zone. The degeneration advances circumferentially and centrally, the leading edge being marked by lipid deposition. Characteristically, the peripheral edge of the degeneration slopes smoothly towards the limbus, whilst the central edge is sharply delineated. The condition is slowly progressive and painless, and not associated with significant inflammatory response, although there is some associated vascularization. Ectasia of the thinned segment leads to irregular astigmatism, and minimal trauma can provoke perforation, in which case tectonic grafting is necessary.

Vitamin A deficiency

Corneal changes in vitamin A deficiency first manifest as corneal xerosis, in which there develops epithelial metaplasia and keratinization, superficial punctate keratitis, mild stromal oedema, and poor wettability of the surface.

Untreated, this progresses to stromal ulceration (Fig. 3.7.8), and, in extreme cases, an acute liquefactive necrosis of the stroma termed keratomalacia develops. There is minimal inflammatory reaction, and perforation often results. Secondary infection is common.

Vitamin A deficiency should be treated with systemic vitamin A supplementation, as well as local measures, such as provision of tear substitutes, topical antibiotics, and topical retinoids to reverse epithelial metaplasia.

Dellen (Fig. 3.7.9)

These are areas of peripheral stromal thinning caused by drying of the cornea. This may be a result of a primary dry eye state, or be a local phenomenon due to tear film disruption by adjacent limbal swelling. This can be caused by muscle surgery, subconjunctival haematoma or other inflammatory processes. The epithelium over the thinned stroma normally remains intact.

Treatment involves provision of lubricants and padding, in association with relief of any precipitating factor, e.g., evacuation of a subconjunctival haematoma.

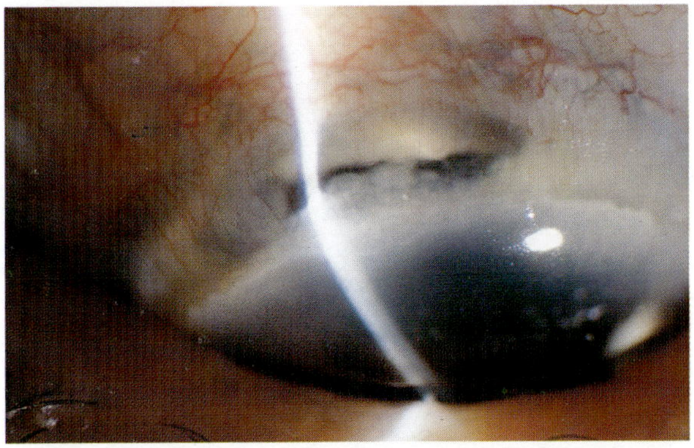

Fig. 3.7.7 Terrien's marginal degeneration.

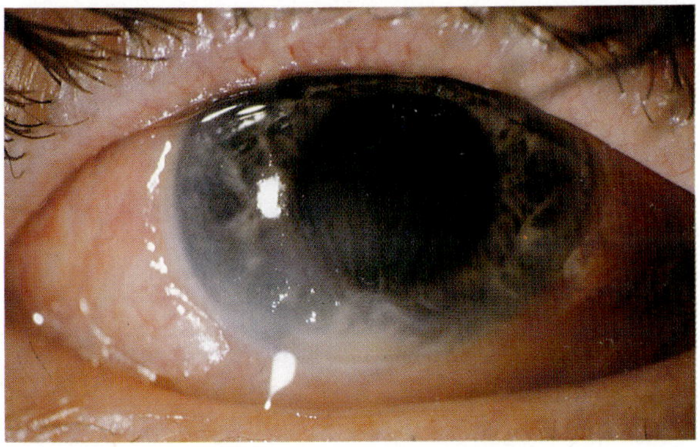

Fig. 3.7.8 Corneal xerosis and ulceration from vitamin A deficiency.

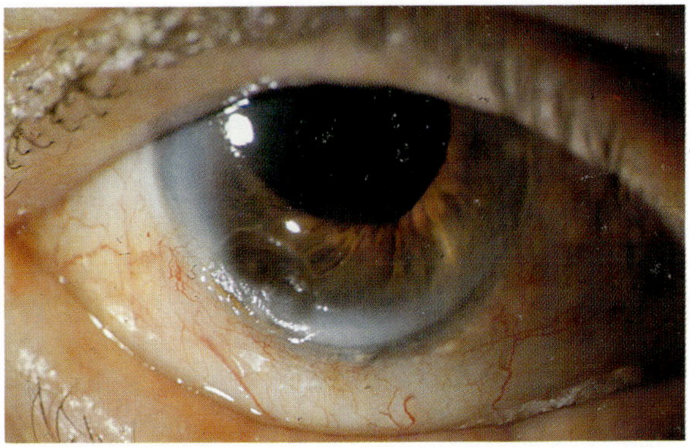

Fig. 3.7.9 Dellen.

CORNEAL DEPOSITIONS

Iron

Deposition of iron in the corneal epithelium is seen in a number of conditions. It occurs in areas of high epithelial turnover, although the precise mechanism remains undefined. It may be related to tear film pooling, or to recurrent epithelial trauma. The source of the iron is unknown, but it is thought to be derived from tears, aqueous or limbal capillary blood or from breakdown of cytochrome enzymes. Histological studies show the stroma and Bowman's layer to be uninvolved.

Hudson–Stähli line (Fig. 3.8.1)

This is a deposition of iron, predominantly in the form of ferritin, which occurs in a horizontal line at the junction of the inferior one-third and superior two-thirds of the cornea (i.e., in the interpalpebral zone). It is a normal physiological feature of the ageing cornea, and is rarely seen in childhood.

Fleischer ring (Fig. 3.8.2)

This is ring-shaped deposition of iron in the corneal epithelium at the base of the 'cone' seen in keratoconus. It is typically not a complete ring, but generally more curved than the deposition seen in the Hudson–Stähli line.

Stocker–Holt line (Fig. 3.8.3)

This is a vertical epithelial iron deposition seen just beyond the corneal edge of a pterygium.

Ferry's line (Fig. 3.8.4)

This line is seen in the epithelium immediately beyond the limit of a filtration bleb after glaucoma surgery. Its shape and position depend on that of the bleb, normally occurring in the superior cornea.

Copper

The deposition of a 2–3 mm wide goldish-brown ring around the limbal cornea at the level of Descemet's membrane is seen in Wilson's disease. It is termed the Kayser–Fleischer ring (Fig. 3.8.5), and is due to excessive circulating copper levels, due to impaired copper excretion and subnormal caeruloplasmin levels.

The progressive disease also leads to tremor, choreiform movements and rigidity when copper is deposited in the corpus striatum. Hepatic and renal involvement is often fatal.

Corneal rings identical in appearance occur in primary biliary cirrhosis and chronic active hepatitis.

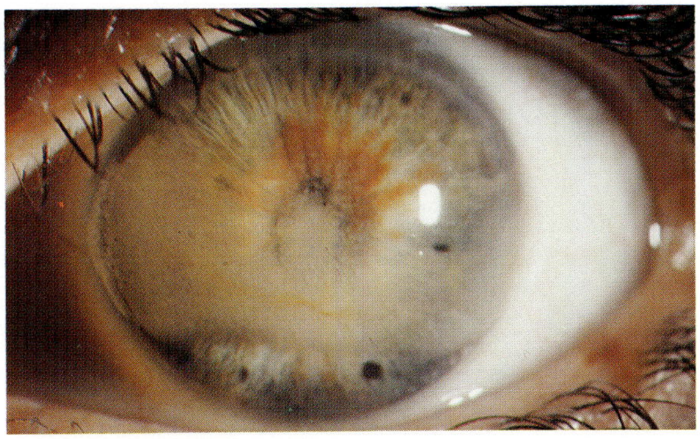

Fig. 3.8.1 Hudson–Stähli line highlighted by co-existing band keratopathy.

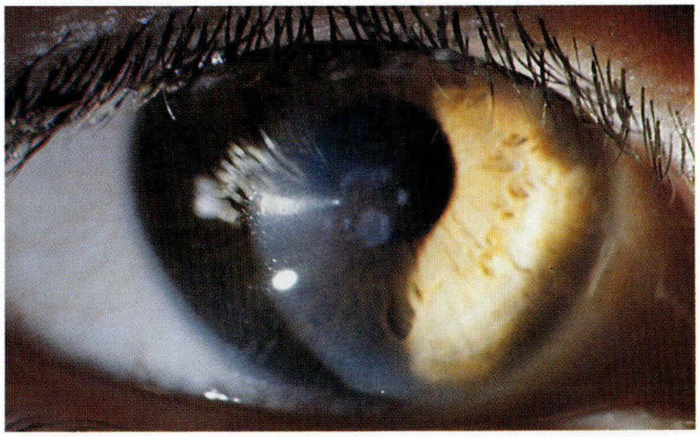

Fig. 3.8.2 (Fleischer ring). Iron deposition around base of cone in keratoconus.

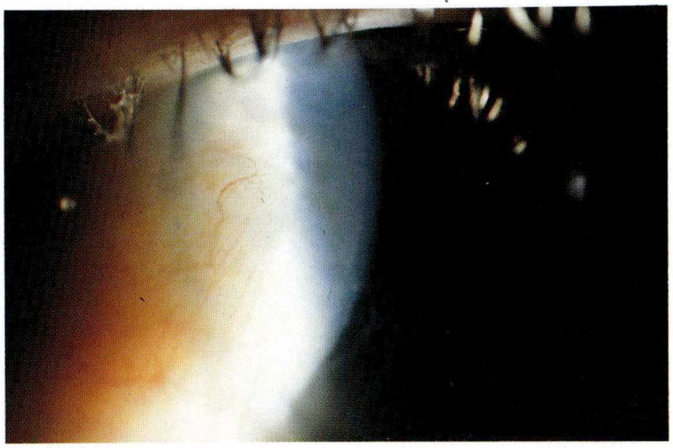

Fig. 3.8.3 Stocker–Holt line. Iron deposition at central edge of pterygium.

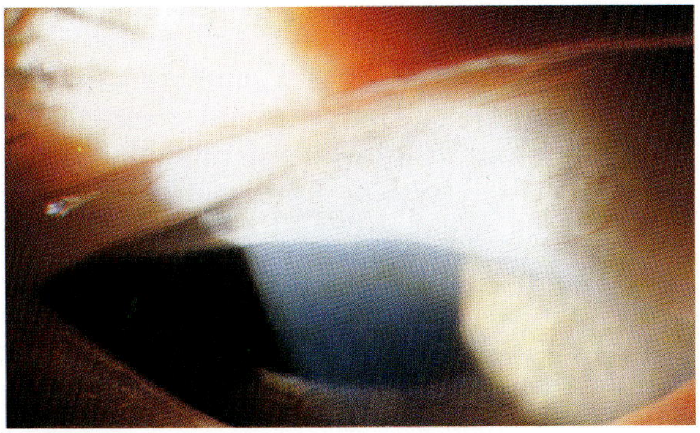

Fig. 3.8.4 Ferry's line at edge of trabeculectomy bleb.

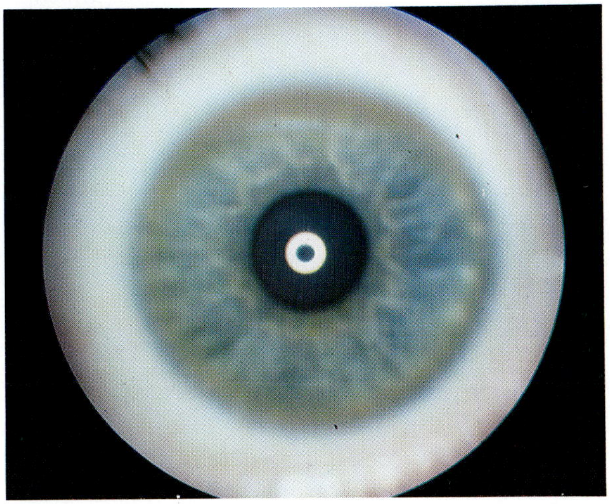

Fig. 3.8.5 Kayser–Fleischer ring.

Drugs

Systemic administration of a number of drugs leads to corneal deposition. 'Cornea verticillata' (Fig. 3.8.6) is a vortex-shaped epithelial deposition due to the formation of complexes between the drug and cellular phospholipids. It is seen following administration of phenothiazines, amiodarone, flecainide and tamoxifen. Cessation of the drug therapy leads to its resolution.

Bismuth, amodiaquine, mepacrine, chloroquine and hydroxychloroquine can also be deposited in the epithelium.

Stromal deposition is seen following treatment with gold-, silver- or mercury-based preparations (Fig. 3.8.7).

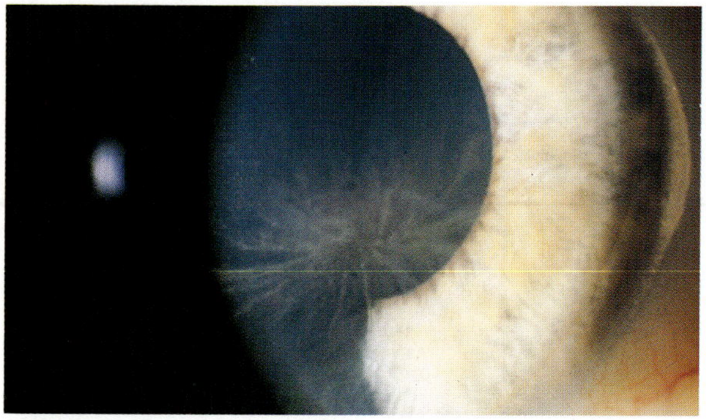

Fig. 3.8.6 Cornea verticillata following amiodarone therapy.

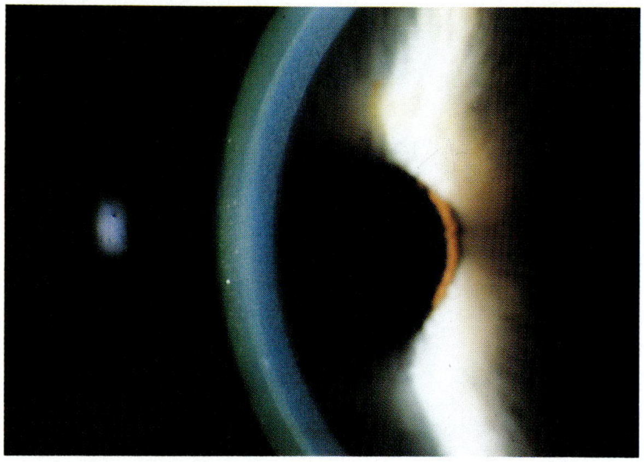

Fig. 3.8.7 Corneal argyrosis.

Fabry's disease

This X-linked disorder is due to a deficiency of α-galactosidase which leads to a deposition of glycosphingolipid in most of the body tissues. Renal involvement may be fatal. The characteristic skin lesion 'angiokeratoma corporis diffusum' consists of clusters of superficial cutaneous dark-red angiectases.

The corneal deposition is in a vortex distribution, indistinguishable from that seen in drug deposition (Fig. 3.8.6). It occurs in asymptomatic female carriers as well as in sufferers. Other ocular changes include tortuosity and aneurysmal dilatations of the conjunctival (Fig. 3.8.8) and retinal vessels.

Arcus senilis (Fig. 3.8.9)

This is a deposition of lipid in the corneal stroma, Bowman's membrane and Descemet's membrane in a ring just within the limbus, and separated from it by a small rim of clear cornea.

Although seen commonly as an involutional change, its onset before the age of 45 may be an indication of hyperlipoproteinaemia. Its depth and size are not related to the severity of any such disorder however. Other features of abnormal lipid metabolism, such as xanthelasma, should be sought, and fasting lipoproteins assayed.

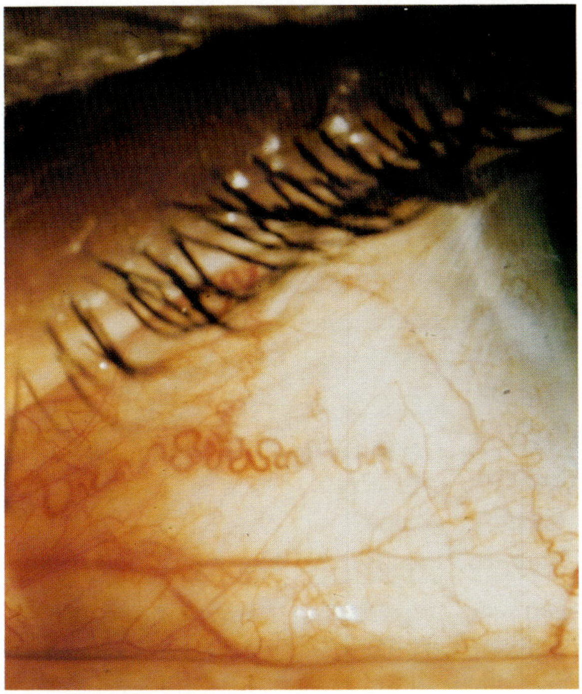

Fig. 3.8.8 Tortuous conjunctival vasculature in Fabry's disease (courtesy of Mr H. E. Willshaw).

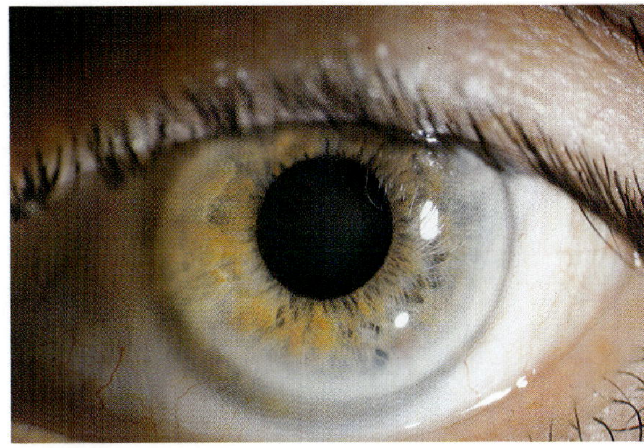

Fig. 3.8.9 Arcus senilis.

Cystinosis (Fig. 3.8.10)

This is a disorder of lysosomal storage, inherited in an autosomal recessive manner, which leads to very high circulating levels of cystine. Deposition of cystine crystals occurs in the kidneys, liver, spleen, bone marrow and ocular tissues.

In the infantile and adolescent forms of the disease, renal failure leads to early demise, but the adult form is not associated with renal involvement.

The corneal appearance is of needle-shaped crystals deposited in the stroma and sometimes a secondary band keratopathy.

Systemic administration of cysteamine stabilizes renal glomerular function but does not influence the corneal appearance. Hourly topical administration of cysteamine is effective in clearing the corneal deposition and improving visual acuity.

Blood (Fig. 3.8.11)

Blood staining of the cornea is a serious complication of persistent hyphaema, particularly when associated with raised intraocular pressure or endothelial damage. The deposition is of haemoglobin and haemosiderin, which begins in the deep stroma, and advances anteriorly. Vision may be severely compromised, necessitating penetrating keratoplasty.

Aggressive medical management of raised intraocular pressure associated with hyphaema, and prompt surgical evacuation of extensive hyphaema which fails to resolve within a few days, minimizes the development of such staining.

Amyloid (Fig. 3.8.12)

Amyloid is an eosinophilic hyaline material which is deposited extracellularly either as part of a systemic disease or locally. Systemic amyloidosis rarely manifests as corneal deposition, which is much more commonly an isolated entity, often secondary to previous ocular disease.

Amyloid shows characteristic histochemical appearances, demonstrating fluorescence on staining with thioflavine-T and birefringence with Congo Red when viewed with a polarizing microscope.

Lattice dystrophy is a localized form of amyloidosis, which occurs as a primary familial dystrophy.

Paraproteins (Fig. 3.8.13)

Deposition of stromal crystals may occur in any of the paraproteinaemias, which include multiple myeloma, Waldenstrom's macroglobulinaemia, heavy chain disease, lymphoma and myeloproliferative diseases, as well as the benign monoclonal gammopathy of unknown significance (MGUS).

The crystals, which are derived from metabolites of the immunoglobulins, can be deposited at any level of the stroma. Their identification should prompt immunoelectrophoretic examination of the serum, since Bence–Jones proteinuria is not invariably present.

Corneal deposits may be sufficiently dense as to require keratoplasty, but recurrence in the graft is not uncommon. Haematological control may be necessary to keep the cornea clear.

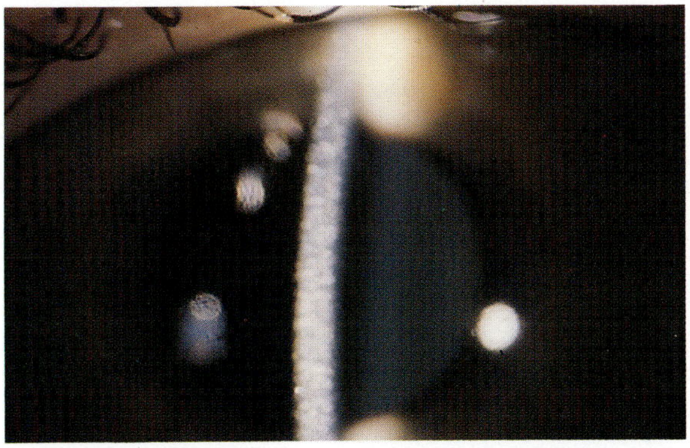

Fig. 3.8.10 Corneal crystals in cystinosis (courtesy of Mr H. E. Willshaw).

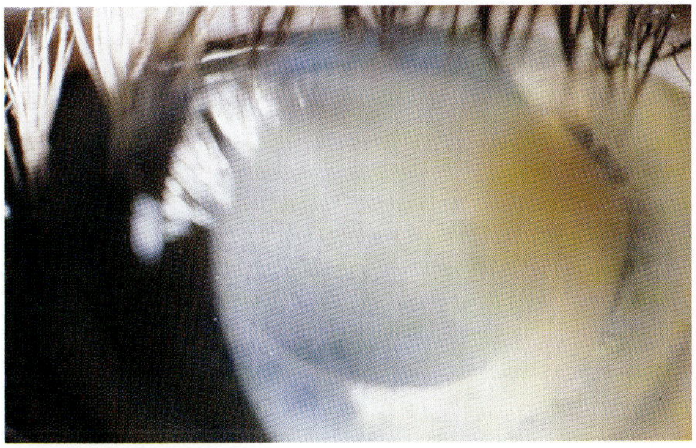

Fig. 3.8.11 Blood staining of the cornea following hyphaema.

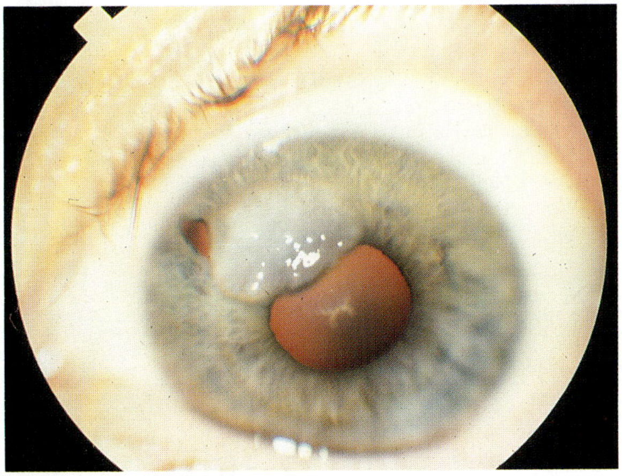

Fig. 3.8.12 Localized corneal amyloidosis following penetrating keratoplasty (courtesy of Mr T. R. Dabbs).

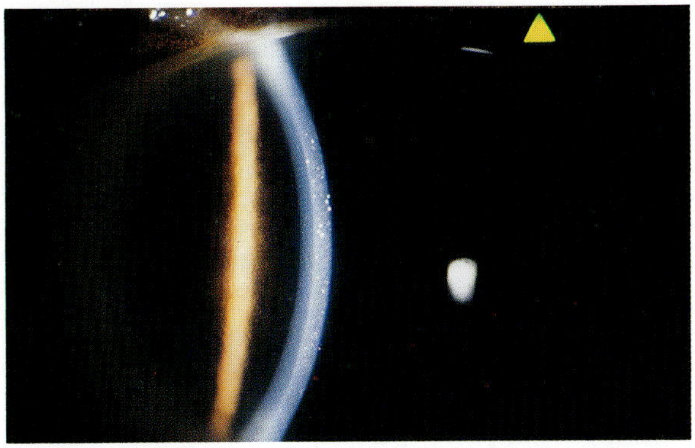

Fig. 3.8.13 Paraprotein crystalline keratopathy (courtesy of Mr A. J. Morrell).

FURTHER READING

General

Casey T A, Mayer D J 1984 Corneal grafting. Principles and practice, 2nd edition. W B Saunders, Philadelphia

Cavanagh D W (ed) 1988 The cornea: transactions of the world congress on the cornea III. Raven Press, New York

Grayson (ed) 1983 Diseases of the cornea, 2nd edition. Mosby, St Louis

Kaufman H E, Barron B A, McDonald M B, Waltman S R (eds) 1988 The cornea. Churchill Livingstone, New York

Smolin G, Thoft R A (eds) 1987 The cornea, 2nd edition. Little Brown, Boston

Anatomy

Hogan M J, Alvarado J A, Weddell J E 1971 Histology of the human eye. W B Saunders, London

Viral keratitis

Darrell R W (ed) 1985 Viral diseases of the eye. Lea and Febiger, Philadelphia

Easty D L (ed) 1985 Virus disease of the eye. Lloyd-Luke, London

Easty D L, Smolin G (eds) 1985 External eye disease. Butterworths, London

Margolis T P, Ostler H B 1990 Treatment of ocular disease in eczema herpeticum. American Journal of Ophthalmology 110: 274–279

Non-viral infective keratitis

Johns K J, O'Day D M 1988 Pharmacologic management of keratomycosis. Survey of Ophthalmology 33: 178–188

Tabbara K F, Hyndiuk R A 1986 Infections of the eye. Little Brown, Boston

Non-infective keratitis

Donzis P B, Mondino B J 1987 Management of noninfectious corneal ulcers. Survey of Ophthalmology 32: 94–110

Nelson J D 1989 Superior limbic keratoconjunctivitis (SLK). Eye 3: 180–189

Tauber J, Sainz de la Maza M, Hoang-Xuan Thanh, Foster S C 1990 An analysis of therapeutic decision making regarding immunosuppressive chemotherapy for peripheral ulcerative keratitis. Cornea 9: 66–73

Watson P G 1990 Vascular changes in peripheral corneal destructive disease. Eye 4: 65–73

Wilson F M, Grayson M, Pieroni D 1973 Corneal changes in ectodermal dysplasia. American Journal of Ophthalmology 75: 17–27

Corneal dystrophies

Bahn C F, Falls H F, Varley G A, Meyer R F, Edelhauser H F, Bourne W M 1984 Classification of corneal endothelial disorders based on neural crest origin. Ophthalmology 91: 558–563

Rodrigues M M, Kruth H S, Krachmer J H, Willis R 1987 Unesterified cholesterol in Schnyders corneal crystalline dystrophy. American Journal of Ophthalmology 104: 157–163

Waring G O III, Rodrigues M M, Laibson P R 1978 Corneal dystrophies I. Dystrophies of the epithelium, Bowman's layer and stroma. Survey of Ophthalmology 23: 71–122

Waring G O III, Rodrigues M M, Laibson P R 1978 Corneal dystrophies II. Endothelial dystrophies. Survey of Ophthalmology 23: 147–168

Ectatic corneal dystrophies

Krachmer J H, Feder R S, Belin M W 1984 Keratoconus and related noninflammatory corneal thinning disorders. Survey of Ophthalmology 28: 293–322

Pouliquen Y 1987 The 1987 Doyne lecture: keratoconus. Eye 1: 1–14

Corneal degenerations

Ansons A M, Atkinson P L 1989 Corneal mosaic patterns — morphology and epidemiology. Eye 3: 811–815

Wood T O 1990 Salzmann's nodular degeneration. Cornea 9: 17–22

Corneal depositions

Bartlett J D, Jaanus S D (eds) 1989 Clinical ocular pharmacology. Butterworths, Boston

Ormerod L D, Collin H B, Dohlman C H et al 1988 Paraproteinemic crystalline keratopathy. Ophthalmology 95: 202–212

Pavan-Langston D, Dunkel E 1990 Handbook of ocular drugs and ocular side effects of systemic drugs. Little Brown, Boston

Rose G E, Lavin M J 1987 The Hudson–Stähli line III: observations on morphology, a critical review of aetiology and a unified theory for the formation of iron lines of the corneal epithelium. Eye 1: 475–479

Scriver C R, Beaudet A L, Sly W S, Valle D (eds) 1989 The metabolic basis of inherited disease, vol II. McGraw Hill, New York

INDEX